Hope, Fears and Wheelchairs *is a powerful exploration of resilience and hope. Tim, a man of deep faith, shares his journey through trauma with courage and a steadfast spirit. As an everyday Kiwi bloke, he brings an authenticity that resonates, showing that healing is possible even in the darkest times. His story exemplifies the mana and strength of character that defines him, guiding others toward hope. Tim's ability to see light amid struggle is inspiring, making this book an uplifting resource for anyone facing life's hardest moments. A compelling testament to faith and human endurance.*

– Cathy Cooney, leader in health and community services

With raw authenticity, humour and pain, underpinned by a confident faith, Tim gives us an incredible insight into living life after losing 92 percent of his body motor functions. While he doesn't underplay the huge consequences of a tragic accident, he writes of a life that pursues new opportunities and actively seeks ways to serve others. I cried. I smiled. I pondered. I praised God. But most of all this book has inspired me to be a better person. Whether you are a support worker, a pastor or chaplain, a health professional, a family member, a neighbour or a friend, you must read this book.

– Charles Hewlett, National Leader, Baptist Union of New Zealand, and author of *Hurting Hope: What parents feel when their children suffer*

Timothy's story is filled with hope and love. Despite suffering a life-changing spinal cord injury, Timothy has been able to adapt to a new normal with the loving and ever-present support of his family, friends and community. Timothy believes God kept him alive to encourage the people around him and to bring hope where possible. The message that rings out is that our sufferings and struggles build resilience, but our character and values are what define us. A comforting and encouraging read for anyone going through tough times, which is all of us at some stage.

– Carolyn Wilson, physiotherapist and senior academic staff member, Toi Ohomai Institute of Technology

In his inspirational book, Timothy shares his experience of life since his traumatic accident in 2010. He writes of not just the challenging times, but of his adventures in life after receiving the diagnosis of tetraplegia, and of his support and advocacy for others also challenged by disability. His infectious enthusiasm for living and how he carved out a life of purpose for himself fill the book, making it a thought-provoking read.

– Gaynor Lincoln, author of *Redemptive Grief*

Hopes, Fears and Wheelchairs

Hopes, Fears and Wheelchairs

A story of faith and hope after the trauma
of a life-threatening accident

TIMOTHY LEE

Hopes, Fears and Wheelchairs
Published by Timothy Lee
with Castle Publishing Ltd
New Zealand

© 2025 Timothy Lee

ISBN 978-0-473-74775-6 (Softcover)
ISBN 978-0-473-74776-3 (ePUB)
ISBN 978-0-473-74777-0 (Kindle)

Editing:
B. & J. Norsworthy
A. Candy

Production & Typesetting:
Andrew Killick
Castle Publishing Services
www.castlepublishing.co.nz

Cover Design:
Paul Smith

Cover Photograph:
Pam Vincent Photography

Scripture quotations, unless otherwise indicated,
are taken from the Holy Bible, New International Version®, NIV®.
Copyright ©1973, 1978, 1984, 2011 by Biblica, Inc.™
Used by permission of Zondervan.
All rights reserved worldwide.

For other versions used,
see the Notes section at the end of this book.

ALL RIGHTS RESERVED

No part of this publication may be reproduced,
stored in a retrieval system, or transmitted
in any form or by any means, electronic, mechanical,
photocopying, recording or otherwise,
without prior written permission from the author.

Contents

Acknowledgements — 9
Preface — 13

Prologue — 17
1. Rich Beginnings and the Call of God — 19
2. When Life Changes in a Flash — 39
3. People Really Do Care — 69
4. Getting the Right Help — 97
5. Finding My Place in an Unfamiliar World — 131
6. Where is God When Bad Things Happen? — 155
7. I'm Broken, But Can I Help You? — 175
8. Channels of Hope from the Weary — 191
9. Sharing the Beauty of 'God's Own' — 207
10. Maybe Tomorrow Isn't So Bad After All! — 219

Notes — 231
About the Author — 242

Acknowledgements

Putting my story into print has been a challenge, given the limitations of my computer software. Overall, it's brilliant and allows me the freedom to navigate websites, undertake research and translate my thoughts into words. However, most days my computer decides that I'm asking too much of it and freezes for several minutes at a time, or the voice recognition function simply disappears off my screen! This means I have to seek the help of whoever is nearby to manually operate the keypad and get me going again; or I nod off to sleep for a few minutes while I'm waiting! On average, this happens several times a day, even more so during the editing process whilst I've had several documents open over two screens.

Thank you to my support workers, family, and friends who have put up with my endless interruptions in this regard. You can see how the practical support of others is vital for me to achieve my goals, not to mention the additional daily help I need with personal cares just to get me up in the morning, drive me to appointments, and put me into bed at night.

Thank you to my wife Jenny, for being there, supporting me on this journey, searching books for page references, checking timelines, and all the while managing my support team, running the household and fulfilling your own vocational demands. You are a faithful trooper, the love of my life, an awesome mother and an ever-present grandmother. You didn't plan on having a husband with such a unique set of needs, yet you have adapted to life with all its new frustrations and demands. Thank you for the example of grace you are to me, and to so many others.

Thank you to my two boys Hamish and Callum, and my precious daughter-in-law Jess, for your willing and faithful support, helping me with practical needs and going beyond the call of duty. The impact of my spinal injury upon your lives has been even more prominent in my mind as I've recounted the events of recent years. You have adapted to a difficult set of family circumstances which has been thrust upon you, and I love you beyond words.

Thank you to my dad and late mum, who have helped to shape my life and endure the heartache of having a son nearly lose his life in tragic circumstances. I am truly grateful for your undying investment in my life, and your example of faithful service to so many over the years. You've stood by my side and given of yourselves without flinching. Thank you to my brother Steve for all your practical help and support. If only I could return the many favours you've extended to our household. Thank you to my sister Trudy who shed tears with me and suffered the shock of my accident in those early days. Your gift of music was a great encouragement to me.

To my friends, work colleagues, fellow parishioners and neighbours – thank you for being there on the journey with me; for your prayers, your generosity, your time, your gifts and your servant hearts.

To those in our precious community who provide an opportunity for me to keep living and serving inasmuch as I am able to – you give back so much to me in return; especially the richness of diversity and culture that broadens my outlook on life. May God richly bless you.

Thank you to Beverley and John Norsworthy for your time and expertise with initial editing in my book, and for directing me with the finer points of authorship. A big thank you also to Andrew Killick and the team at Castle for your guidance and patience with me in the process. My thanks to Andrea Candy, for your editing prowess, and generosity with me as a newbie!

Thank you to John Douglas, my faithful supervisor through the thick and thin of pastoral ministry. And a final thank you to the late Martyn Norrie who provided the impetus and encouragement for me to pursue the task of putting my story into print. You have left a footprint of great worth to so many, and it was a great privilege for me to journey with you through such a debilitating illness, not to mention the intrusion into your plans for retirement.

Preface

Over the years, people have suggested that I put my story into book form. My initial reaction was to dismiss the idea. I reasoned that it wouldn't be a big seller, that I was too busy, and lacked the energy to make it happen. As time moved on, I couldn't ignore the sense that I had a significant and unique contribution to make, one that I trust will encourage, broaden, and enhance the reader's life.

I consider myself to be just an ordinary Kiwi bloke with some training and life experience under my belt. I'm certainly not the fount of all knowledge and theology but, as a preacher, I'm privileged to open the Scriptures and encourage people on their journey of life and faith. Over time, I've been presented with other unique opportunities to teach, motivate and inspire. I'm compelled to respond if the things I've learned and experienced can make a positive impact on the wellbeing of others.

I'm proud to have grown up in this beautiful land of Aotearoa and I celebrate the cultural diversity of our nation. It's a privilege to connect with a range of people from different cultures in our local community, the wider Bay of Plenty, and beyond; not only those in the disability sector, but people like you and me who struggle with a whole gamut of challenges that life presents.

I have tetraplegia (synonymous with quadriplegia) which is defined as the inability to move upper and lower parts of the body, including breathing muscles. According to the New Zealand Spinal Cord Injury Registry, there were 157 individuals with a traumatic spinal cord injury in 2024, which translates to 29 per million, or 0.00293 percent of 5,356,700, as the population was then. Biking injuries have consistently been in the top two sporting causes of SCI in NZ since registry records began in 2016, the other being water-based leisure/sporting activities. Seventy-five percent of bike sporting injuries have been through mountain biking.[1]

I'm okay with having tetraplegia despite being a minority statistic, because I'm confident enough in my own skin and still able to use my God-given gifts to contribute to society. What I'm not okay with is been labelled a tetraplegic. You may ask, "What's the difference, Timothy?" I generally point out that we don't usually go around saying, "There goes Andrew the blind man, Vivian the haemophiliac, Bob the alcoholic, or Susan the Buddhist." So why should I be described by my condition?

Tetraplegia is visibly obvious and certainly gets people's attention in public, but it doesn't define me. The things that define me are primarily my character, the values I hold dear, and the cultural heritage that was passed down to me. What is sometimes less obvious, whether you have a disability or not, are the invisible disabilities that many of us wrestle with; things like depression, grief, loneliness, anxiety and fear. These things can affect our ability to function, relate with others, and navigate the world around us. That's true for me too, but they shouldn't be the signpost on my forehead as well! Living with tetraplegia has its ongoing frustrations and grief, yet there are broader challenges which we all have to contend with in these uncertain times, such as rising inflation, climate change, the rippling effect of wars in Ukraine and Gaza, and the significant impact on health as a result of Covid-19. And let's not forget the mental health challenges which affect one fifth (20 percent) of our population, according to the World Health Organisation's wellbeing statistics, posted after Auckland's second lockdown in March 2021.[2]

I believe there is a loving God who identifies with our brokenness and loss, giving us hope for tomorrow. I've learnt both a practical and a prophetic trade in this journey of life. By that I mean I'm a mechanic and a preacher. I hope the following anecdotes and reflections will be an encouragement and inspiration for you as you chart your journey of life. I'm trusting that God's voice will be the loudest from within these pages.

This book is for you if you've suffered a traumatic event in life; if you're living with a disability of some kind; if you're wrestling with mental health; if grief and loss are a reality for you; if you've ever had to battle ACC; if you wonder how brokenness and healing can live in tension with each other; if you question where God is in the midst of suffering; if you lack hope and direction in life; if diversity and belonging are important values to you; or if you need to laugh on a bad day.

I have included a few questions at the end of each chapter. These are designed for personal reflection or could be used in a group setting. We all have a story to tell. Making sense of that will enable each of us to invest in others' lives and illustrate the things we've learned from our own journey.

Prologue

Monday 31 May, 2010, dawned clear, if a little brisk. I was keen to go for a mountain bike ride to blow away the cobwebs on my day off, and it was a perfect day for it.

Physical exercise in a beautiful location was guaranteed to do wonders for my health and wellbeing. I kept a pretty busy schedule as the senior pastor of Rotorua Baptist Church and as my weeks culminated in fulfilling but energy-taxing Sundays, I found Mondays the best day to relax and change focus.

At age 44, I wasn't a competitive rider, but thoroughly enjoyed the thrill of navigating most tracks, even if I was not the fastest rider around. I had begun mountain biking approximately six years earlier in the pine forest on the lower slopes of the Tararua ranges in the Horowhenua, close to Levin township where we lived then.

I was prepared to take some risks in the hope of improving my skill level, even if I had the odd tumble; a regular event in this particular sport! That said, I tended to avoid the big jumps, leaving those to the more fearless and youthful, like our then teenaged son Hamish, who had become quite proficient within a very short time of riding the tracks in Rotorua.

Hamish was at school that day of course, so I gave my neighbour Wilfred Wong-Toi a call to see if he wanted to join me. He was a keen mountain biker and also took Monday afternoons off from his busy job as an ear, nose and throat surgeon. We had been neighbours for a year, but this was the first time we had ridden together, as we were both usually quite busy in our respective vocations.

As we set out that afternoon, riding from home, I thought how fortunate we were to live only minutes from the Redwoods Whakarewarewa Forest Park – just 'The Redwoods' to us locals. It was a paradise on our doorstep, a playground for anybody into mountain biking, jogging, walking, horse riding, or exercising the dog. I was looking forward to switching off and concentrating solely on the enjoyment of an afternoon ride. I was just shy of two years into my ministry, the church was growing, we felt settled as a family, and life was generally ticking along nicely.

The trees were magnificent in the sunshine that day and track conditions were ideal, dry enough to maintain a good speed, but not too dusty. But once in the bush, we had to concentrate; there is a very small margin for error in this sport, as experienced mountain bike riders will know.

Most of the ride was uneventful. I was just glad to be out in the fresh air, enjoying my brand-new GT Force mountain bike. It was performing well, and I felt I was too!

Near the end of our ride, we had to negotiate the exit trail where there were two options to enter the last downhill section. One was narrow and rutty; the other had a 'drop-off' which required a level of gumption to tackle. My new bike gave me a fresh dose of confidence, so I decided to take the latter track.

This was the third time I had entered that jump. The first time, I fell and laughed about it; the second time, I negotiated it successfully. This time, as I approached the jump, I knew I would need a fair bit of speed in order to clear the drop. I started pedalling harder...

Chapter 1

Rich Beginnings and the Call of God

The search for discovering our purpose in life starts when we are very young and continues throughout our lives.
– Pastor Tom Holtey[1]

I was born in Pukekohe and grew up as a farm boy. When Mum and Dad were sharemilking we lived on a dairy farm in Drury, South Auckland. Then they bought a farm further south in the heart of the Waikato. We were situated near the end of the school bus run on Paratu Road in the Richmond Downs/Walton area. Matamata, Cambridge, Morrinsville and Hamilton were not far away as the crow flies.

Along with my younger brother Stephen and sister Trudy, I initially went to nearby Walton Primary School, then on to Matamata Intermediate and College. I was a fairly average student, although I excelled in athletics and played hockey as a winter sport. The farm was a great environment to maintain fitness for these activities.

I'm often reminded how enjoyable farm life was growing up back in the 1970s and 1980s, when I look at one of my uncle John's paintings, which hangs proudly on our dining room wall (picture 1). Dad is in the foreground of this rural scene, feeding out hay from the back of his tractor. He would hop on and off the tractor just-in-time to steer it away from fences and gullies. Our dog called 'Yuk' is in the paddock nearby.

In the middle ground of the painting is our cowshed, farm orchard and silage pit. This reminds me of milking cows and eating tart Granny Smith apples while wandering through the orchard with my friends (and trying to avoid the codling moth larvae in the apple cores). We were often making our way toward the fun experiences of swinging from the twisted supplejack vines in the nearby native bush, shooting rabbits or making huts in the hay barn.

Our house and garage feature in the background with the surrounding trees and greenery. Home was a welcoming environment, warmed by an open fire in the lounge during winter, the place where I was encouraged to practise playing the piano for relatives. When I was young, our house had ancient features like a wringer washing machine and a dial-up telephone which was on a party line connected to our nearest neighbours. When the phone rang, we had to listen carefully to see if it was our specific ring sequence. There's a blast from the past that makes me feel old!

In front of the house was the veggie garden, where corn on the cob, beetroot and beans grew in abundance. So there was always enough food for everyone. Visitors would come and go, from relatives staying at Christmas time, to people who needed pastoral support from Mum and Dad. It didn't matter what time of day or night, or if we were celebrating as a family, everyone was made to feel welcome. We would often have folk on the fringes home for lunch after church on Sundays. By that, I mean those who would sometimes come alone or were maybe not the easiest people to entertain. By extending the hand of fellowship, Mum and Dad taught us to be generous and hospitable, showing care for people without any sense of partiality, thereby instilling principles of leadership that would reap benefits later on in my life.

Our parents also modelled a strong work ethic, whether it was from the disciplines of stock management and maintaining farm equipment, or simply through doing the hard yards of summer harvesting. I loved hay season – watching the neighbour cut the long grass in the early mornings while Dad milked the cows, learning to condition the hay while sitting on the tractor's mudguard alongside Dad, working late into the evenings to stack the barn, and taking breaks to enjoy food brought to us by Mum.

Of course, there were other disciplines we learnt during these formative years. Mum and Dad weren't afraid to give us a smack for being disobedient (totally illegal now!) It was all good character-building stuff. They also used the natural consequences of our actions as our teacher as well. For example, there was the time when I was treating the farm motorbike like a motocross bike, going over jumps and ruts which gave the frame and suspension a hard time. I learnt the hard way by falling off and landing in the mud, or when the frame broke and needed repairing at the shop. I had to push it home from the back of the farm that day!

Beside the house in the painting is the garage, with a room on the end where I slept on a saggy old wire-wove bed alongside the other single bed where my model railroad sat. I moved out to the garage in my early teens. It was a brave move away from the main house but all part of learning to be independent. Dad built an extra bay onto the garage one year, and it was long enough that we could have a homemade table tennis table down one end. On the end was a small covered lean-to, split in half; one side for firewood, and the other for coal. It was only a short walk across the front garden to a small external door beside the chimney where we stored enough wood and coal to feed the fire on winter evenings.

I enjoyed splitting firewood, and Dad let me chop down some of our gum trees one year, filling up several trailer loads of split firewood to sell. I made a few bucks, but it probably cost Dad in fuel to deliver them. Any opportunity to earn some pocket money meant I could save a few dollars to spend on family holidays, put toward my model railroad, or waste on sweets!

As a young teenager I joined a hay gang with a couple of neighbours. I earned enough money picking up hay over several summers to buy items like a car stereo for our farm car. It was an old Škoda, also featured alongside the garage in the painting. It wasn't exactly a top-shelf brand in those days, but that didn't bother me as it effectively became my first car! I drove it to school sometimes so I could stay late for hockey practices or athletics and participate in Saturday sports without needing a lift from Mum and Dad. There were benefits to getting a licence as soon as I turned 15! It was also handy to drive my brother and me to youth group events associated with Morrinsville Baptist, and when I began working, I used it to travel to and from town.

I didn't have a clue what I wanted to do career-wise, but nearing the end of my Sixth Form (Year 12), I was offered an apprenticeship in heavy equipment automotive engineering at Maber Motors Morrinsville (now Power Farming Holdings Ltd). To this day, it remains one of the largest agricultural farm machinery outlet and service departments in the southern hemisphere and is now the wholesale distributor for Deutz Fhar tractors in Australia, New Zealand and the United States.

I worked as a diesel mechanic, servicing tractors mostly, but the company had a large variety of farm machinery brands at the time, so I gained wide and varied experience in the agricultural industry. In the first year of my apprenticeship, my boss said, "Here's a van, you're on field service now!" I felt reticent initially, still gaining confidence as a mechanic. However, I learnt to solve problems; adapt on-the-fly if I was short of a particular tool; relate with farmers who were tricky customers; read the service manual even if it was a last thought at times; and to pray when all else failed!

Field service meant travelling huge distances at times, from east coast to west coast, and from as far north as Mangawhai Heads, to the Tongariro Prison Farm south of Lake Taupō. I also loved going to the annual National Fieldays at Mystery Creek near Hamilton. Maber Motors had a stand there each year and we got free tickets if I asked the salesman to put some aside for me. I reminisce over those days with a collection of 1/32 scale model tractors which I display in the garage. Alas, some things don't change – big boys and their little toys!

I suppose I became a bit of a petrolhead as well, attending car shows and motor racing events, enjoying any opportunity to get behind the wheel. I know that Mum and Dad had a few concerns for my safety as a young risk-taker who was still learning to read the road, observe other motorists, and be responsible for other passengers. This was evidenced when they received a phone call from me one night. My brother and I were on our way home from a youth group event and I lost control on a bend, crashing through a farm fence and into a paddock. We were fine, but that was the end of the Škoda!

I eventually bought a Mark II 1600 GT Ford Cortina from a workmate. This was a much more desirable car amongst my peers! I had lots of fun with that car, for example, going for a two-week holiday up north with my mate Andrew Harris. We had both completed the first year of our apprenticeships, Andrew in building and joinery, me as a mechanic. I had roof racks which I used to secure my skis in the wintertime. They allowed us to mount a kayak on top, and we had just enough room to fit a surfboard inside. We had a pup tent and all the basics for camping, like a gas cooker. It was a great opportunity to celebrate the rigours of working full-time as two young mates, with no agenda except to stop and camp at whatever beach we felt like exploring.

I'm convinced that angels were watching over me and keeping me safe in my younger years. I ended up being involved in a few car crashes as a passenger; add to that the farm incidents like falling off the motorbike or off the back of a trailer-load of haybales. I even got knocked off the top of a truck load of hay by a telephone wire which hit me in the mouth as we were travelling down a farmer's track late at night. Somewhat dazed, I shook myself off and sprinted after the truck, hoping that my mate who was driving would hear my shouts before he turned onto the road and left me behind!

I was very active outdoors, enjoying tramping with friends or jogging across the paddocks of our farm in order to improve my fitness as a young athlete. I could waterski, and relished opportunities offered to me by friends whose families had boats. My mate and I always had enough sports equipment in our car boots to enjoy Sunday afternoons with friends at a park or the beach. We would grab anything we could to erect a volleyball net, kick a ball around or fly a kite. These memories are precious to me.

I also learnt to snow ski on Mount Ruapehu as a young teenager. It became a real passion of mine during the winter months.

I skied most of the commercial fields in the North and South Island, rating Treble Cone ski field near Wānaka as the best New Zealand has to offer.

I still like attending the Banff Mountain Film Festival, which showcases the world's best mountain films from more than 40 countries. They usually schedule a showing during wintertime in Rotorua. There are a lot of people in our community who are into outdoor sports such as mountain biking, river rafting and skiing. Many hundreds turn out to this annual event in Rotorua and I sit there, the only individual in a wheelchair amidst a sea of able-bodied adventure junkies, still able to enjoy short films of people mountaineering, extreme skiing, and surfing the world's largest waves.

It was during my time as a young adult attending the Morrinsville Baptist Church that I sensed a strong call to pastoral ministry. We had a large and flourishing youth ministry where I was given the opportunity to lead at a young age whilst attending weekly social events, monthly Youth for Christ rallies at Founders Theatre in Hamilton, and Easter camps at Finlay Park, Lake Karāpiro near Cambridge. This put me in good stead for the future. Not only that, but the pastoral needs of others profoundly impacted my vision and dreams for the future.

The incident that has stuck in my mind the most was when I observed a mum looking after four children on her own at a youth event one evening. After receiving my next pay packet, I was compelled to purchase some groceries for her. I believe that God was sowing seeds of love and compassion within me, especially for people living in needy circumstances. As Martin Luther said,

Since, however a true Christian lives and labours on earth not

for himself but for his neighbour, therefore the whole spirit of his life compels him to do even that which he needs not do, but which is profitable and necessary for his neighbour.[2]

My desire to help and work with people full-time was so strong that I wanted to leave my work as a mechanic immediately. But God had other ideas! Through prayer, advice from Mum and Dad, and trusted mentors, I sensed that God wanted me to wait. I subsequently spent the next 10 years continuing to work as a mechanic until I knew it was the right time to venture into theological studies.

I look back and see the prime value of this 'waiting' time as an opportunity to critique the world, learn more about leadership, understand in depth what life is like for the average New Zealander, and to consider how best to respond when faced with the genuine needs of others. After all, what good was I in pastoral ministry unless I could identify with my fellow Kiwis doing life in the trenches of a constantly evolving society and having to wrestle with all manner of struggles unique to our culture? Not only that, but I needed to understand what it really means to be compassionate, the essence of which is 'to suffer with', derived from the Latin root word *compati*.

In 1986, Jenny (then Thompson) moved into the area to take up her first teaching post at Te Aroha College. Jenny began attending Morrinsville Baptist Church where my family had worshipped for many years. Together, we became part of an effective leadership team, both enjoying working with young people, but catching an eye for each other at the same time. We fell in love and married on 26 August 1989 after a short engagement. Our wedding had to fit in with school holidays as Jenny was teaching in a three-term school year then.

We spent the first 18 months of our married life staying in a rented farmhouse down No. 7 Road, Springdale. It was central to work and church for both of us. We look back with fond memories on those early years of developing and growing together as a couple. During this time, we saved enough money to embark on an overseas trip, buying a return ticket for 12 months. Who does that these days?

We headed off to the United Kingdom via Hawaii and Los Angeles, enjoying things like Disneyland and a day trip to the city of Tijuana in northern Mexico. We met up with Jenny's brother Geoff and sister Suzi in London, bought a Volkswagen Combi van and travelled extensively throughout Europe for 10 weeks, visiting France, Spain, Italy, Austria, Switzerland, Germany, Belgium, and the Netherlands. Greece and Turkey were out of reach by road due to civil conflict in Yugoslavia.

We had a wonderful sense of freedom, stopping to sleep at random spots beside the road, or to grab decent showers at the occasional campground. It was hot, but we managed to explore many landmarks. Some were unplanned, like arriving in Le Mans when the famous 24-hour race was on and seeing Barcelona before the 1992 Summer Olympics. At that time, we were able to watch a bullfight. I knew about matadors, but I wasn't aware of the gruesome way they killed the bulls with multiple swords. Bullfights were later banned in some parts of Spain.

We arrived in East Germany not long after the Berlin Wall came down. The contrast to the West was very apparent. We had to use a hand pump to refuel our van, for example. I enjoyed seeing the super yachts in Monte Carlo on the French Riviera and swimming in the crystal-clear waters of the Mediterranean. We climbed the Eiffel Tower, visited the leaning Tower of Pisa, and Le Mont-Saint-Michel where the tide rushes in and out faster than a galloping horse. Of course, we made important stops at the Mercedes-Benz museum and factory in Stuttgart, plus the BMW Museum in Munich; lots of drooling over expensive motorcars!

On a more sombre note, we visited a concentration camp in Dachau, arriving to see a memorial wall laden with human bones. Inside were many images of the atrocities committed on the Jews at the hand of Hitler. We made our way through a field where the remains of barracks lay and at the far end of the enclosure, we had the opportunity to enter the gas chambers. My emotions were somewhat numb at the time; it's hard to describe this experience with words that give sufficient respect to what happened during the Holocaust.

Arriving back in London, we found work and stayed for a further eight months. Initially, I worked as a security guard on what was then the old Financial Times building in central London; now, it's the Industrial Bank of Japan's head office for Europe, right next to St Paul's Cathedral and close to the River Thames. Later, I worked briefly for a diesel specialist working on a variety of trucks and buses, followed by a job with an automatic transmission specialist, fixing London taxis.

Some mornings, when winter was at its peak, I would leave for work in the dark, travel on the Tube, and arrive home in the dark. On one occasion, Jenny's brother Geoff took great delight in jumping out from behind a brick wall to frighten me as I made my way down the footpath near the place where we were staying at the time. I nearly throttled him before calming down from this alarming experience!

I was hoping it would snow during Christmas, but alas, we only had a brief dusting one night which didn't settle for long.

We did enjoy a Christmas dinner with Kiwi friends and, of course, saw the Tower of London and all the royal pageantry that London has to offer.

We ventured on several Tiki Tours to Ireland and Wales during that time. Jenny's brother Geoff and I even travelled over to the Isle of Man and watched the famous Tourist Trophy (TT) motorbike racing, where riders travel at phenomenal speeds through narrow village streets and picturesque rural lanes. At one point, Jenny's parents came out from New Zealand and joined us on a brief trip to Scotland – that was fun. We travelled as far north as Inverness and I took a photo of the Loch Ness monster, albeit a concrete one on the edge of the lake!

The van broke down on numerous occasions in our travels, but we had a few tools and enough Kiwi ingenuity to get by, whether it was in Spain, Germany or Scotland. On one occasion, we were having issues starting the van and I had to remove the starter motor in a supermarket carpark. I was able to solder broken wires back together using a nail which I heated up at a nearby petrol station. Other examples were replacing brake shoes and resetting the float level on the carburettor, all on the side of the road! I also recall when the windscreen wipers stopped working during heavy rain in Milan. We tied bailing twine to the arms and looped it around through the front doors, leaving the windows just open enough to manually move the twine from left to right to operate the wiper arms. It was hilarious, but effective!

On one adventure, Geoff and I travelled to Switzerland for a ski trip. This will always be one of my lifetime highlights. To get there, we embarked on a 24-hour bus trip from London to the Lauterbrunnen Valley in the Jungfrau region of Switzerland (picture 2). You could ski all day and not be on the same slope twice. We rode what was, at that time, the longest cable car in the world and accessed the ski slopes each day via a cog railway up the hill, passing exclusive mountainside villages like Wengen where royalty stayed for their ski holidays.

It was my first experience of skiing in deep powder snow in contrast to being on top of the piste. I fell over on one occasion and had to search for some time to find one of my skis! I even skied down from the Schilthorn summit (2,970 metres) which is in the Bernese Alps, looking over from the valley where we stayed. This was the location where James Bond (Roger Moore) skied down from the restaurant at the top in the 1969 movie *On Her Majesty's Secret Service*. At least I didn't have men firing machine guns at me as I made my descent!

At the end of our OE (overseas experience), Jenny and I visited a missionary friend in northern Thailand en route back to NZ. First, we stayed for a couple of days in Bangkok and took in some of the city sights. I recall visiting the restaurant across the road from our hotel. They served a small dessert which consisted of mangoes and sticky sweet rice. It was so nice that I had to wander over there several times for more!

Then we flew north to the city of Chiang Mai, visiting an animal park where we rode on an elephant and attended a snake show. We were glad to be sitting in the back row away from the mat when the performers tipped out a basket of snakes and gathered them up just before the snakes entered the seating area!

Our friend Judith met us, and we drove north beyond Chiang Rai up to her village where she served amongst the Hmong people with Overseas Missionary Fellowship (now OMF). It was very humbling to stay in her hut, sleeping with mosquito nets and making bread out of flour which we had to sift the weevils out of beforehand! I recall digging a hole in the ground outside one day in order to mix some concrete and repair her steps to the front door. Several local people turned up to help without me asking. One chap was clearly high from smoking opium which was readily available! Nonetheless, we got the job done, albeit at a slower pace than I would have hoped.

Near the end of our stay with Judith, we visited a remote mountain village which was about an hour's drive away. On arrival, we attended a church service with the local people, after which a family invited us to lunch. We entered a room which had a small table in the middle and limited seating around the outside. They presented a flat plate with a large quantity of white rice piled on top, and a cup filled with bamboo shoots alongside. It was very generous hospitality, given the poor status of the local people there. While we ate, a dog ran around the table flicking its tail which had a weeping sore. We were especially glad that we had had our vaccination jabs before leaving London!

Enduring the hot weather was a good dose of Third World context for us. We even managed to bring Swiss chocolate all the way home via the United Kingdom. Naturally, it was very carefully wrapped up in our travel bags during our two-week stay in Thailand! It was somewhat deformed by the time we came to eat it, but still quite delicious.

On reflection, we consider it an absolute privilege to have travelled for a whole year. I could tell many more stories. We prayed and seriously wondered whether God was leading us into ministry overseas at some stage, as Jenny's parents had been missionaries in Bolivia when she was young. Visiting Thailand was an opportunity to test the waters, but it was very clear to us once we were back home that New Zealand was where God intended us to be.

Before we left the United Kingdom, I had sent my CV back to different firms in the Kapiti Coast and Horowhenua districts north of Wellington. It was always going to be easy for Jenny to pick up a job, with her skills as a secondary school teacher, and the demand for diesel mechanics gave me confidence about my work prospects. So, we thought we would look at changing location. The owner of a small agricultural business in Levin wrote to me just before we left the United Kingdom with the possibility of a job and suggested I contact him on return to New Zealand. They ran a farm machinery and lawnmower outlet in Levin.

We arrived back in New Zealand in May 1992. Within a week, I was offered my old job back in Morrinsville and several other opportunities, including a variety of jobs with different tractor firms – even one managing a bull farm. But the calling to pastoral ministry was still tugging away at the back of my mind, despite the ease of remaining in the industry as a diesel mechanic. There was still a pull to stay in the Waikato, as our friends and my rural roots were there. However, after careful consideration and prayer, we decided to leave the Waikato and venture south. At that stage, my mum and dad were 'across the ditch' in the South Island town of Motueka northwest of Nelson. They offered us a place to stay for a month or so until I commenced work in Levin at Rowell Farm Equipment, the company which had offered me a job when I left the United Kingdom.

Jenny ended up picking up work at both colleges in Levin in her capacity as a secondary school teacher. Her family, who lived in Upper Hutt, had a bach in Raumati, north of Wellington. We were privileged to be able to stay in it for several months and commute up to Levin for work. Whilst there, we enjoyed regular visits to Jenny's family who were nearby on the coast and in Wellington. It served us well for several months until we rented a home in Levin. We stayed in that house for 12 months before purchasing our first home in July 1993.

These were precious times when we were relatively free of commitments outside of work. I skied the most I ever had during the first few winter months, travelling up to Mount Ruapehu every two or three weekends a month on average. In addition to that, I enjoyed working on some of my practical projects, like building a go-kart, developing my model railroad and embarking on house renovations. This was a new season for us, the birthplace of our two boys Hamish and Callum, the establishing of new friendships, and the launchpad of my ministry as a pastor.

We became involved at Levin Baptist, and it wasn't long before I began working with the young people through a ministry of the church. The group grew and flourished until I was appointed to a part-time position as the youth pastor in 1997. After that 10-year period of travelling and working as a mechanic, God opened the door, and we had a real peace that the time was right to fulfil my desire to commence working with people full-time.

I knew I needed some theological grounding, however. While I seriously considered full-time study, it would have meant moving to Auckland. So we decided that I should pick up the Youth Internship Diploma at the Bible College of New Zealand's (BCNZ, now Laidlaw College) campus in Palmerston North. This was more appropriate for our family at the time. After I completed my diploma, Levin Baptist asked me to become the sole pastor. So I changed hats, as it were, and we employed a youth pastor to maintain the work I'd developed with the local young people.

Being exposed to the rigours of full-time pastoral ministry was not an easy change. However, I grew and learnt a lot in the years that followed. It was really hard work leading what was a very theologically conservative church through some difficult years of change. I was glad to have the support of David McChesney who was senior pastor at Palmerston North Baptist Church at the time. Hugh Kemp, who had been my dean at BCNZ, became my supervisor and a great source of wisdom and support as well. He and his wife Karen remain friends to this day, each of us seeking to make a difference for the wellbeing and spiritual health of our fellow Kiwis in our own respective contexts.

The church grew as we focused our efforts on children's ministry, eventually employing a children's worker to invest in this area and broaden Levin Baptist's service to the local community. Jenny became the chairperson and licensee of the early childhood centre Levin Baptist Kindy and Care as it was then (now Levin Baptist Kindergarten) which was associated with the church. Both our boys went through this thriving and valued early childhood facility. It had a great reputation amongst local families and bolstered our relationships within the community. We also made some initial changes to the church building complex and, with a vision for the future, set about planning to develop the main auditorium to accommodate growth.

My practice was to arrive at work early and set the coffee machine percolating, thus sending the smell of Irish cream wafting through the building. How can you work without good coffee! Sometimes I joined the kindy staff for morning tea. Much of my time was invested in sermon preparation, leadership responsibilities, and pastoral work, although I also enjoyed playing squash, working on house renovations, and activities with the boys.

Our sons attended different primary schools which suited their developing personalities, and recreational and learning needs. We formed some strong friendships as a family, remaining connected to locals there like Alan and Jill Baldwin, the Clappertons, Kerrs, Christiansens, and Pearces, to name a few. We retain a close connection with Adrienne Kerr who formed a strong bond with our boys and was a leader amongst her peers in the youth group.

We gathered this group together weekly on a Sunday evening and were blessed by the hospitality of Adrienne's parents Ross and Sally at their home in town. They were always willing to help with social events, especially when it came to tramping which was their passion as a family. We eventually employed Adrienne in a part-time youth capacity, and together with her elder sister Bronwyn, I ran a group for the students at Horowhenua College. We called it CHAOS, which stood for Christian Happenings At Our School. I worked closely with one of the teachers from a rural family where, as it happens, I had previously serviced their farm tractor. Adrienne eventually married David Brewerton which was a special ceremony for me to facilitate. They ended up naming their eldest son Jethro Timothy after me! This will always be a special honour for me to carry in this connection with their family.

It warms my heart to think of the special relationships we formed in Levin. It was a great context for our boys to grow spiritually and have fun in the early years of their lives. My good friends Neil Watson and Alan Baldwin were fellow leaders in the Levin Baptist Boys' Club which we developed from its former status as a Boys' Brigade group. Neil eventually moved to Rotorua and remains one of my closest friends to this day.

As usual, the boys got involved with school activities, soccer, swimming, paper runs, and the like. We enjoyed being close to the ocean, often ending up on Sunday afternoons at Waikawa Beach just 20 minutes' drive south of us (picture 3). A special aunty died during this time and left us some money in her will. So we commissioned a local artist who did pastels to draw the boys at that beach. To this day, those portraits sit proudly on our dining room walls. The boys' cousins Jono and his sister Megan lived at Waikawa Beach, along with their adopted parents Andy and Karen Chaplow. Sadly, Andy dropped dead suddenly while working as a teacher aide at Manakau Primary School. It was a sad time, but drew us all closer together, as we remain to this day.

Eventually, God began to loosen our roots in Levin, and it became clear that it was time to move on. So I sent my CV to the Baptist Union and engaged in several interviews in the months that followed. To cut a long story short, we moved to Rotorua in August 2008 where I took up the position of senior pastor at Rotorua Baptist Church (RBC).

It was a big call to uplift the boys and shift to a different location, particularly for Callum who had been diagnosed with autism at the age of three. We had to leave our familiar surroundings where he had well-established routines and knew people with whom he was comfortable. Since that time, we have upskilled ourselves as parents, seeking to accommodate his unique needs and provide an environment where he can thrive as much as possible.

In the early days, we attended a pilot course called Tips for Autism. We learned an enormous amount, so when they advertised for more facilitators, Jenny applied. The facilitators at that time suggested that she would be an ideal candidate. Effectively, she contracted to the Ministry of Education (MOE) in this job and remained with the company for 13 years. She loved the work, travelling anywhere from as far north as Kaitāia, to Oamaru down south.

As parents of a child with neurodivergent needs, we became acutely aware that anything outside of Callum's familiar routine was a challenge for him. Spur-of-the-moment activities still tend to throw him off balance. So, right from when he was young, Jenny and I learnt the strategy of telling him about up-and-coming events well in advance – whether in the next hour, the next day or even in a month's time. This gives him time to process what might happen, to prepare for any implications, and to identify any new individuals with whom he may have to interact.

There have been unique challenges in parenting Callum, not the least of which has been to mitigate any decline in his mental health. Despite that, he has grown and matured over the years, learning to adapt and strategise for himself. We are super-proud of him, his caring nature, his generosity toward friends, and his freedom to converse with us openly about anything – sometimes too openly!

Though it took some time, I'm happy to say that both Callum and Hamish settled and adapted well to life at Rotorua. It wasn't easy for us to leave our friends and the good people of Levin Baptist Church after almost 12 years' pastoral ministry there. When we left, I felt like I'd abandoned the people there, but we knew it was right to move on. Such is the bond you form with parishioners and locals as a pastor.

Jenny had served in several different teaching roles at the colleges in Levin, forming strong friendships with colleagues, some of which still remain today. Along with her passion for early childhood education and attending to the growing and unique needs of our son Callum, she also launched a new career in professional development as an autism educator.

Levin will always be the place where our boys were shaped in the younger years of their lives, and where I transitioned from automotive engineering to cutting my teeth as a pastoral leader.

Questions for reflection:

When it comes time to move on, how do you weigh up what doors might be closing, and when new ones are opening at the same time?

What gives your family hope? How does our New Zealand context enhance that hope?

How do you include your family in your journey of vocational change?

Do you have a clear sense of calling or purpose in your life? Is there a faith element to it? What help and guidance could you access to clarify this?

Chapter 2

When Life Changes in a Flash

When suddenly you seem to lose all you thought you had gained, do not despair. You must expect setbacks and regressions. Don't say to yourself, "All is lost. I have to start all over again." This is not true. What you have gained you have gained... When you return to the road, you return to the place where you left it, not to where you started.
– Henri Nouwen[1]

...The next thing I knew was waking up down a dirt bank, immediately aware that I couldn't move at all. It was clear that I'd had a serious fall off my mountain bike, and my head was in a rather uncomfortable position, propped up against the stump of a punga fern. I was in pain and could feel blood dripping down the corner of my eye.

Strangely, I didn't panic, and I can honestly say that I had a sense of peace, which I acknowledge could only be God. I prayed the first thing that came into my mind: "Whatever is happening, God, I want You to get the glory." I haven't recounted this often because I don't want to sound pious, but that's the fact of it.

My neighbour, Wilfred, was ahead of me so he hadn't seen me fall. It occurred to me that he was probably at the bottom of the downhill section by now, wondering where I was. Some minutes passed and I was very glad when he came back up the track and found me.

The next person who came along was an off-duty fireman. Who better to be first on the scene than an ENT surgeon with specialist knowledge of the head and a member of emergency services with local knowledge of the forest! I believe this was the providence of God, rather than some random coincidence.

Though the memory of the impact still eludes me, I learnt later that I had gone over the handlebars and headfirst into the sharp edge of a tree which may have been milled. Wilfred rang the hospital to prepare the Emergency Department (ED), and he contacted Jenny. I can't imagine her shock and the myriad of thoughts that must have been going through her mind.

Jenny's story
It was late afternoon, and I was starting to prepare dinner when Wilfred called from the forest. It was a quick phone call, just telling me where Tim was and that he'd had an accident. Wilfred didn't give me any details, and simply requested that I meet him at ED.

A range of thoughts rushed through my head; one was remembering our friend Keith who had recently spent a couple of nights in hospital after a mountain bike fall. So I prepared an overnight bag for Tim and rushed down to the hospital. I had checked with our son Hamish (aged 15) that he was okay to keep an eye on Callum (aged 13). I didn't want the boys to feel they were a low priority, so I attended to their most immediate needs and made sure they felt settled and cared for before I set off for the hospital about an hour after Wilfred's call.

Callum's autism means that dramatic events create a challenging, new dimension, given the complex lens from which he views life. Tim had asked him earlier in the day if he wanted to do something together that afternoon, but he was happy doing his own thing. Even today, he beats himself up about this at times, feeling in some way that he was responsible for Tim's accident, and that it could have been avoided if he had chosen to spend time with Tim instead. I can't begin to describe the tension or burden this has been for him, particularly in the early years.

As I made my way towards ED, I still felt very much in the dark about what had happened to Tim. Feelings of anxiety arose within me when I noticed a helicopter taking off from the helipad; I wondered if Tim had been taken away due to a serious injury before I had even seen him. However, at ED I was told that the ambulance hadn't even arrived yet! I was sent down to the entrance and told to wait. While I wasn't thinking the worst, I was a bit jittery with butterflies in my stomach.

Then Tim arrived. He looked very grubby with blood and dirt all over his face, but he was talking to everyone (typical Tim!) This gave me instant hope. They got him settled and I was allowed in for a quick "Hello". All he kept saying was, "I'm sorry, I'm so sorry!" I told him that I loved him and we said a quick prayer together.

One of the ED staff sent me out into the hallway again, saying it was serious, and that they needed to work on him. They asked if there was someone I could contact to be with me. I thought of our friends Keith and Julie Turner. Julie, a nurse, would understand the medical side, and Keith could help organise whoever needed to be contacted.

It was now 6.30pm and I was keen to have my family there. I knew from previous tragic family incidents that my dad Brian Thompson, a former policeman, was very practical and pragmatic when responding to similar situations. He and Mum

(Mary) lived in Upper Hutt, but I rang them anyway and asked if they would come. Dad said, "Yes," straight away. Knowing they would come as soon as possible instantly lifted a burden. Ringing loved ones and telling them about the accident was incredibly hard – especially when I didn't know much myself. In the end Mum and Dad stayed six weeks with the boys. We so appreciated them and their willingness to drop everything and come to Rotorua.

Keith must have contacted the elders at church. It wasn't long before the relatives' room in ED began to fill with people. I felt so loved and supported. Jason our youth pastor, who'd become really close to Tim, was so upset! I just cried and hugged him. I didn't have any words.

When the consultant told us the prognosis, I just felt numb: Tim could easily die. They were worried about infection from the dirt in his head wound. So the first step was to take him to surgery to clean up and stitch his head – a five-hour operation! We heard later that Tim had an enormous amount of the forest floor in his head wound. They had to scrub it out with a hard brush.

The people working that night were our neighbours: Stephan Neff, the anaesthetist, and Wilfred Wong-Toi, the ENT surgeon. Chris Ngar from church, an orthopaedic surgeon, also joined in. These were all people that we knew and appreciated. God is good.

By 9pm, the intensive care unit (ICU) was full of our friends and family, all waiting for Tim to come out of surgery. Most folk from the Baptist Church had become aware of Tim's accident by now, and many of them turned up to ED along with folk from other churches. We were spilling out everywhere. Friends of ours from church who run a local restaurant and catering business turned up with trays of baking for everyone. Tim's parents David and Beth Lee had arrived earlier from Tauranga to be with our boys. Later in the evening, Helen Ritchie, a friend from church who lived nearby, popped home to relieve them so they could come to the hospital. I was so thankful for the hospital's open-door policy as I felt very supported by having friends and family around.

At the same time, I was overwhelmed, having to play the 'pastor's wife' role. I can't tell you how wonderful it was to see my sister Suzi and her son Stan arrive from Auckland. She instantly took over and become the 'gatekeeper' – she had the right manner for the role. I felt that I could just be me and relax with her.

Tim was back from surgery about 11pm. He was not a very pretty sight, but it was Tim, and he was alive. Stephan (the anaesthetist) then outlined the situation to the whānau. He didn't make any promises but said, "If Tim does survive, he could be on a ventilator for the rest of his life." That was very sobering news.

By now, I was even more numb and unsettled. There was nothing left to do but wait and see, so the hospital staff encouraged us to go home and sleep. We dragged ourselves away and left Tim to their care. Arriving home, we were greeted by a note from Hamish telling us where everyone could sleep – he had signed off as 'hotel manager'. His thoughtfulness that night still makes me smile. I couldn't sleep in our bed as it was such a reminder of the empty space, so I 'slept' in our study.

The next morning, it was so lovely to get up and just sit around chatting together with everyone over breakfast. You don't know how important family is until times like this hit. They accept you for who you are. There isn't the expectation that you have to be strong and supportive of others.

The ICU staff had handed us what was left of Tim's attire. I didn't want to see it. Tim's helmet was completely split in two. Brian said it was like someone had taken to it with an axe. Dad later visited the site of Tim's accident. It was very clear that if he hadn't been wearing a helmet, he would have been in a much worse state, possibly not here with us at all.

Having finished breakfast and freshened up, we made our way to the hospital to meet the doctors responsible for Tim's care. They explained the situation in detail and Suzi translated the medical jargon for me. Tim needed specialist help for his face, eye and neck, which meant he needed to be transferred to Middlemore Hospital in Auckland. The picture they painted was pretty bleak, especially in relation to the spinal injury.

Their plan was to keep Tim comfortable and sedated until he could be transferred to Middlemore via a fixed wing aircraft later in the day. Unfortunately, the weather didn't allow for that. So, on Wednesday they got the Westpac rescue helicopter down from Auckland to enable him to be transferred safely.

As the days passed in Auckland, there were so many things that made life easier for me. Firstly, I stayed at my sister Suzi's place in Shelly Bay, Howick, not far from Middlemore Hospital. It was fantastic to feel so comfortable and surrounded by love in her house instead of staying in a motel by myself.

The beach was only a short distance away and provided solace for me as I walked amongst the driftwood and shells in the mornings. I was able to begin processing what was happening, surrounded by the sea, the bush, and the neighbouring farmland of Whitford. I would often go off for an hour's walk, spending the early minutes of the day just 'defragging' and releasing a myriad of feelings.

There were some days in Shelly Bay when I cried for the

whole walk. Other days I put on my headphones and listened to music. I would regularly play songs on repeat, like 'Praise You in This Storm' by Casting Crowns. The words, "You never left my side and though my heart is torn, I will praise you in this storm,"[2] were a great comfort for me.

Another tool that helped me process what was happening was my journal. I found that writing down the thoughts in my head was very cathartic. As noted from research by Callie Koziol, "Psychologists advocate that journalling can become a dynamic tool for personal growth and healing."[3]

Mornings were also an opportunity for me to make phone calls. It became clear that I needed to get a book in which I could record and keep track of all the organisational details and decisions I had to make.

Tim's story

As the paramedic secured an oxygen mask over my head, I remember thinking, "This isn't normal." Members of the fire brigade stretchered me out of the bush to a waiting ambulance. I recall the creaks and bumps in the vehicle as we made our way back to the road. Ambulances aren't exactly limousines!

I was certainly not a pretty sight for Jenny to see that day, when she did not yet know the extent of my injuries (pictures 4 & 5)! I had sustained a flexion injury or incomplete spinal impairment between C_4 and C_5 vertebrae, several vertebrae were cracked, my nose was broken, spinal fluid was leaking out of my nostrils, my jaw was dislocated, I had scalped my head, and the socket beneath my eye had sunk into my face. One eye was dislodged so my eyesight was compromised. Life is mostly not sustainable with a spinal injury from C_2 vertebrae upward, so you can see how close I was to leaving planet Earth that day.

The complexity of my injuries meant several specialist physicians were involved in the surgery that night. There was a huge risk of infection, and my life hung in the balance. Not many people can say that two of their neighbours helped save their life! Stephan recalls plucking pine needles out of my skull while other physicians worked on me. Along with Stephan and Wilfred, I'm also grateful to Dr Chris Ngar, a former parishioner at RBC, who followed my progress and helped us interpret the medical prognosis in the months that followed.

The first I knew of visitors in ED was when regaining consciousness after surgery. I was heavily sedated, though strangely aware of familiar voices in the hallway next to my room. I recall hallucinating a few times. In the first instance, I imagined being strapped to a contraption that moved in all four directions simultaneously – presumably some kind of rehabilitative bed that doesn't even exist!

On another occasion up at Middlemore Hospital, I thought the staff were trying to get me to sleep one night, feeding me more and more drugs while hiding behind the wall and saying something like, "We'll knock him out eventually!" Another time, I imagined that a technician came to repair our TV on a stormy night. In my 'memory', he climbed up through the ceiling of ICU and onto the roof to fix the aerial where he discovered a couple of staff members getting up to no good. These visions were quite vivid, but hard case given that ICU is on the ground floor!

When I left Rotorua Hospital for the flight to Auckland, they reduced my sedation briefly, allowing Jenny enough time to communicate with me before take-off. I blinked to acknowledge her. They told Jenny it was a risky flight, given my fragile state. Though I didn't know it at the time, friends Keith Turner, Jason Mikaere, Helen Ramsdale, and Ann Pascoe (née Fletcher) were present to support Jenny and pray for me while they saw me off on the helicopter (picture 6).

Keith took a couple of photos which Jenny wasn't keen on initially. He convinced her to keep a record, saying, "Tim is going to be okay, and these pictures will be a testimony in your story." It's a strange feeling to see those photos now, with all the life-support machines strapped to my bed, and friends standing arm-in-arm alongside Jenny. Even though I've told this story many times now, my emotions have caught me off guard again as I write and recall the people involved on the day of my accident. I'm eternally grateful for their support.

By Wednesday evening, word had spread to our wider Baptist family and other members of our community. Kelvyn Fairhall (head accountant for the Baptist Union at the time, and former trustee of our family trust) met me on arrival at Middlemore Hospital and prayed for me. It was also a blessing to have family connections with the orthopaedic surgeons, which made my treatment much more streamlined.

Once they reduced my sedation level, I was able to communicate by blinking with the medical staff. Their communication with me was all very calm and professional. I recall something going on with my throat. My best guess is that they were removing an intubation device before carrying out a tracheotomy.

After the surgery to reconstruct my skull, I was placed in a coma to allow my body some respite from shock. Given the impact to my frontal lobe, the physicians were concerned that there could be significant brain damage. I was in a coma for 10 days altogether and spent a total of 40 days and 40 nights in intensive care (ICU). It was touch and go, but after several attempts in the ensuing days, they managed to bring me out of the coma.

Readers familiar with the biblical narrative will recall identical periods when God's people had to wait and endure tough times. For example, it rained 40 days and 40 nights for Noah in the ark; Moses was up Mount Sinai for 40 days when God gave him the Ten Commandments; Jesus fasted for 40 days and 40 nights before commencing His ministry and mission amongst the people. So, 40 days is quite symbolic of being tested on the journey of life and faith, as I've experienced firsthand.

It became clear to me at the time that the major focus of ICU was to enable patients to breathe on their own – nothing else! I had an intubation tube at first, until they installed a tracheostomy in my throat through which to breathe. I had a stomach peg for feeding, and a 'suprapubic' catheter tube in the lower abdomen to drain my bladder and help reduce infections. The surgeon who installed it had to perform the procedure twice as the first one failed. He was a bit distracted because he was working on another patient and training someone at the same time. This didn't inspire a lot of confidence! I feel for those who have had more significant detrimental implications to their health as a result of medical misadventure.

Over time, physicians were able to perform several less invasive procedures on me without the need for a local anaesthetic, because I couldn't (and still can't) feel anything from my upper chest down. That said, if you squeeze my skin too hard or pull the hairs on my legs, I can feel it. Mum did the same thing to me when I was a nipper if I misbehaved in church! Of course, *that* didn't happen very often!

We have billions of neural pathways in our body. An incomplete spinal injury means that some nerves are alive, in contrast to a complete spinal injury where the spinal cord has been severed. Having some live nerves means that I have a tiny bit of movement in my arms and legs, fingers and toes. This is a good thing in terms of what the physiotherapist can work with to help improve function. However, the downside is that I can feel nerve pain, particularly in my legs.

On one occasion in ICU, the pain was so excruciating I went into a foetal position on my bed. That's no small effort, given my lack of trunk control and inability to move my arms and legs. I found out later that the critical care staff debated over the best medication to reduce my pain. They ended up giving me ketamine, which is mostly administered in the early stages following a serious accident or trauma to the body. In sufficient doses, it is strong enough to sedate a horse. It's possible they gave me a stronger dose than necessary. It took the pain away but knocked me out in the process! I still vividly remember vomiting the moment I woke up. I could easily have choked but received instant attention from the nurses. These nurses provide excellent care and do 12-hour shifts, one nurse per patient.

I was treated well in ICU, apart from one grumpy nurse whom I would best describe as 'old-school'. On one occasion, she disturbed some of the bed set-up of the guy next to me, without consulting him, while he was away having some treatment. Bear in mind that if you don't have the right mattress, with memory foam or air pumps to stimulate your circulation, there is risk of pressure areas, or bedsores.

Once, a couple of nurses were working with me and the old-school nurse came along, saying, "Don't worry about that; he doesn't need it." I was so afraid of her that I asked the critical care doctor assigned to me to pull some strings so she would never be rostered on to help me again. Whatever the doctor did, it worked, and I was so relieved!

I was interviewed later at the spinal unit about my experience in ICU. That nurse was definitely a topic of conversation, and I learnt later that she received disciplinary measures for her behaviour. Of course, there were some really nice nurses, and I took great delight when they were rostered on with me. Never underestimate the power of a decent bedside manner! Generally, I received very good care and still hold a great deal of faith in the healthcare that Kiwis are offered here in New Zealand from critical care staff across the board.

It wasn't all bad in ICU. Visits from family and friends were a huge emotional boost for me during the six weeks I spent there.

Jenny and Suzi visited regularly, and Jenny's parents brought the boys up from Rotorua for several weekend visits. Staff allowed them to visit after midday and only two at a time. To enter the ward, you had to go through two locked doors. This was so different from Rotorua's open-door policy. The boys shared with me what they were up to at school and then usually passed the time playing on their phones while Jenny read books. It was so nice just having them there despite my not being able to communicate properly with them.

It was important that both boys received some counselling later on to help them process my accident. As it happened, Callum had started on anti-anxiety medication three weeks beforehand. Many of these medications take about three weeks to become effective, so the timing was great. God works in amazing ways! We were blessed to have a special psychiatric nurse, Kaylene Buckley, from the Infant, Child and Adolescent Mental Health Service (ICAMHS) who spent considerable time helping Callum. She became his close friend and confidante, helping him interpret an event which was not easy for anyone to deal with, let alone someone with special needs. Kaylene is one of many individuals for whom we are eternally grateful to have travelled the journey with Callum.

My uncle John, an artist, created two paintings for me. While they are now framed and sitting proudly on our walls at home, they sat beside my bed and brightened up the space during those bleak days in Middlemore Hospital.

I remember my sister Trudy smuggled her piano keyboard in one evening as well. I think the therapeutic nature of music convinced the staff to let her bring such a large musical instrument into the ward. Trudy sang and played familiar Christian songs. Family and staff all joined in, and my emotions got the better of me, tears streaming down my face. I desperately missed church and singing with my spiritual family. Bear in mind that I still had a tracheostomy (I had it for four weeks in total) so it was very difficult to speak, let alone sing. Some would say it was a good thing that I couldn't perform either function!

My brother Steve and our parents visited regularly. My dad was an expert at relieving nerve pain in my legs by stretching them up to a vertical position. The nursing staff didn't have time to indulge me with such pleasures. None of my medications gave the relief that this simple stretch achieved. Steve talked about all the usual stuff of daily life, and together with family he encouraged me through words, prayers and anecdotes. I could tell that Steve and Trudy were feeling the pain of this life-changing event with me. Elizabeth Watson aptly said, "I know that we live in the lives of those we touch."[4]

My family continues to be a faithful and bolstering factor in my life. Dad describes how he and Mum would often cry in the car going home to Tauranga after each visit with me. Mum died in 2015 after wrestling with dementia for years. Being a loving and supportive mum was the thing she cherished most in life.

She struggled with her own identity, finding failure and shortcomings in her intellect. That didn't mean a thing to us kids growing up because she was so caring, providing the nurture we needed to navigate the early years of our lives. While we will never know, both Dad and I have sometimes wondered if my accident accelerated the dementia and its crippling effect on her cognitive ability.

Something that I found particularly frustrating in ICU was the staff for whom English was a second language (ESL). I distinctly remember what felt like a small leak in the tracheostomy tube bearing down on my upper chest on one occasion. The tube gave me a gentle but regulated source of oxygen. I tried so hard, with my raspy throat, to convey what was wrong. At times like this, the combination of specialist equipment associated with my tracheostomy and ESL nurses who couldn't work out what I was saying created just too big a gap in understanding and addressing my needs.

On a brighter note, I was able to watch the All Blacks and an occasional movie on the TV which happened to be near my bed. Nothing like some distraction on the box, as we say! Little things like this can make all the difference to patients in long-term care in hospital. And food often becomes all-important!

In Middlemore ICU, they had some delicious frozen yoghurt ice creams which gave relief to my dry mouth, which was probably the result of the concoction of medications I was taking. Of course, I was reliant on the nurses to hold the ice cream for me. I could suck on a piece of ice which helped as well. There was risk of choking if the ice went down the back of my throat because I had no way of clearing it. The nurses were very careful but gave me opportunity to try when I was up for it.

I remember the day the doctor removed my tracheostomy

after slowly weaning me off life-support. He immediately put his finger over the hole in my throat. Then I could talk – what a relief! Being the spiritual person that I am, the first thing I said was, "I'd love a cream liqueur!"

This particular critical care doctor was renowned for wearing Magnum PI-type shirts covered in flowers. He was a top bloke, always injecting humour into the conversation, yet, at the same time reassuring me that my breathing would be okay. He had to be very careful choosing the right day to remove the tube from my throat because it wasn't a case of shoving it back in straightaway if I couldn't sustain breathing on my own. They would have to sedate me and perform another tracheotomy, presumably creating access by making a new hole in my throat.

I still have the lasting scars that remind me of early intervention for survival, both physical and emotional. The words of the song 'Scars' by a band called I Am They seem apt:

Darkest water and deepest pain
I wouldn't trade it for anything
'Cause my brokenness brought me to you
And these wounds are a story you'll use
So I'm thankful for the scars
'Cause without them I wouldn't know your heart
And I know they'll always tell of who you are
So forever I am thankful for the scars.[5]

Jesus Christ bore the scars of crucifixion beyond His resurrection from the dead, showing them to His closest disciples as evidence of the cruel and ancient punishment He endured. Though it's not easy to comprehend, I believe Jesus Christ was fully divine, yet He became fully human on our behalf and therefore He can relate to all we experience in life, especially the hard times, as I can testify.

> *He was despised and rejected – a man of sorrows, acquainted with deepest grief. We turned our backs on Him and looked the other way. He was despised and we did not care. Yet, it was our weaknesses He carried; it was our sorrows that weighed Him down.* (Isaiah 53:3-4a, NLT)

At times I felt alone and anxious in ICU. I recall an elderly Samoan woman who cleaned the floors. She came alongside me on one occasion, put her hand on my shoulder and said, "Timothy, God hasn't finished with you yet!" It felt like God was speaking to me directly. He is like a heavenly father to me. I can't fully describe how this felt. It was surreal, but it lifted my spirits and made me feel not so alone anymore. I'm convinced she was a real angel, but I never saw her again.

> *For He will command His angels concerning you to guard you in all your ways. On their hands they will bear you up, so you will not dash your foot against a stone.* (Psalm 91:11-12, NRSV)

I was encouraged by visitors and the many messages of support, both locally and even from overseas. It was humbling to think that my family and I could be the object of such warmth and compassion from many different contexts. If I'm honest, I was struggling in my own self as reality began to sink in: "God, why am I here?" I was finding it difficult to trust the God whom I worship in the midst of my circumstances and told Him in no uncertain terms that it was "just not fair!" In the biblical account, Job stated,

Today my complaint is bitter; his hand is heavy in spite of my groaning. (Job 23:2)

I imagine that's like being under a ruck with the ex-All Black Nepo Laulala's foot pressing down on your head – not a pleasant place to be!

I encounter many who, like myself, get rattled, become angry or complain about the tough and irreconcilable things of life. They question the existence of God or wonder what His intentions might be. Job certainly did, but he remained resolute in trusting God despite the grief and loss that he endured. Trusting in something or someone greater than ourselves is a virtue, yet many of us fall short because pride makes us want to stick it out on our own. All the while, I believe God is in the wings waiting for us to call on Him for help. After all, He's got broad shoulders!

You may have heard of the man who fell off the edge of a cliff. He managed to grab the branch of an overhanging tree. Hanging on for dear life, he called out, "Is anyone there?"

There was no response, so he called out again, "Is anyone there?"

The reply came: "I'm God and I'm here, you can trust me."

The man said, "What should I do, God?"

"Just let go."

After a pause, the man said, "Is anyone else there?"

Fifteen years on, I will be the first to admit that trusting God is hard. Perhaps one of the inconceivable realities of my tragedy is that I'm limited to banging my head on the pillow in response some evenings and expressing my anger toward God. Yet, I truly believe that God hasn't abandoned me, nor was my accident His fault. He's given me the freedom to act any way I like, and hasn't reneged on His promises, despite my doubts and fears in this journey. I will address the topics of suffering and injustice in Chapter 6.

About halfway through my stay in ICU, Jenny and Suzi gave me the news that I would most likely never walk again. My immediate response was to say, "I'm content with that so long as I can still preach." Miraculously, I still can! I guess they came with fear and trembling that day, not knowing if I would fall apart on the spot or perhaps retreat into myself.

Most patients transition from ICU to the high dependency unit (HDU). I went straight to the orthopaedic ward and stayed there for a further four weeks. Our friends the Powleys came to visit one day. Rob brought his daughter Alayna as she had been recording some music in Auckland. She is a local identity in Rotorua and has the sweetest voice, which I liken to Brooke Fraser's (New Zealand singer-songwriter). Rob often accompanies her with a guitar. He is a legend himself, a faithful music teacher for many years, and as lead guitarist, an integral part of our church music team at RBC. I recall bursting into tears the moment they left, a measure of how precious it was to have friends show their care for me in the best way they knew how, with the power of music.

Whilst in the orthopaedic ward, I was dealing with a significant pressure sore on the back of my head due to the bracing used in ICU to support my head. Unfortunately, they didn't monitor the condition of my skin underneath the brace well enough, and I needed a skin graft. It took about six months to heal. I couldn't wait to get out of Middlemore Hospital, having heard that a bed might open up for me at the spinal unit in Otara. At least I could receive more visitors than in Middlemore, I reasoned.

On one occasion, I was fortunate that the nurses relaxed

their rules and allowed my mate Andrew Harris (affectionately known to me as 'Butch') to join me after visiting hours and watch the All Blacks play on TV. I had to pay for a TV in the orthopaedic ward, but that was a small price to pay for the pleasure it gave me during treatment.

Butch is a faithful friend who came to see me regularly. He usually arrived with his wife Vanessa's trademark fruit sponge, covered with custard and still warm. We would sit outside my room facing the evening sunsets over Auckland. There was a roughcast wall in front of my room with a galvanised pipe for a handrail. Butch would place my heels on the bar so I could stretch my legs while we ate our pudding together and talked about his latest house renovation project. That was a really nice stretch, relieving some of the nerve discomfort and swelling in my legs while we enjoyed the space together. These were very special times.

I'm no different from any other person with a spinal injury, having to mitigate perennial problems like pressure sores by altering my position regularly. At Middlemore Hospital, the nurses would wake me up every two to three hours. This was frustrating to say the least, especially when they woke me up during the most valuable rapid eye movement sleep. I had to negotiate getting longer periods of sleep before they woke me up and rolled me onto a different side.

These days, I manage pressure sores by alternating the side I sleep on. If I'm feeling negative, I sometimes roll my eyes when asked by Jenny or one of my support workers which side I would like to sleep on. My response is: "This is what my life consists of now!" However, with a sophisticated memory foam mattress and under the careful eye of my diligent support workers, I manage to keep pretty good skin integrity.

Pressure sores can develop within hours, either in the lower sacrum area of the back, or on the heels or toes, and they can take months to heal, as I know from experience. I'm grateful that, unlike other acquaintances with spinal injuries who have been on bedrest, going on in excess of three to four years now, I haven't had sores that became gaping holes, requiring surgery and prolonged medical intervention. Sorry to be so graphic! I'm not usually one to discuss the intricacies of physiology in such detail if I can avoid it. But this is reality, folks, and I've learnt to call a spade a spade rather than 'a digging instrument', as I used to when Jenny and I first got married.

On arrival at the spinal unit I was assigned a vast amount of support – a neurologist, physiotherapist, occupational therapist, registered nurse, dietician, urologist, social worker, and even a counsellor. What does a pastor need a counsellor for? Well, pastors need counsellors at times, just like anybody else. They help us process the deepest things that trouble us and prevent us from living each day with a sense of wellbeing. We can let worry and anxiety become much greater factors than they should be. It's no surprise that mental health problems are on the rise. Don't get me wrong; I have my bad days and have to pick myself up and carry on like the rest of us. But I've learnt how to respond to the tough days and endure suffering, with more beneficial outcomes for myself and the people on this journey with me. (More on this in Chapters 6 and 7.)

Once I was settled at the spinal unit, Jenny returned to Rotorua to care for the boys. Her sister Suzi's home in Auckland was a wonderful retreat for Jenny during those early hospital stays for me. We are also grateful to Brian and Mary who stayed with the boys while Jenny was in Auckland. They continued to be faithful supporters and prayer warriors over the years.

Rehab life at the spinal unit in South Auckland had its own routines. After taking what seemed like forever to get up in the morning, we eventually got breakfast delivered from Middlemore Hospital, about four kilometres away. We couldn't bank on hot bacon and eggs by the time it had travelled that far through Auckland traffic! I did encounter one nurse in the last week of my stay at the spinal unit who wanted to argue the toss when I asked him to microwave my dinner. I'm not going to get food poisoning from heating up my food; I want it hot, thank you very much!

Hospital food had very few highlights for me. They often served nachos *under* the mince so they were soggy by the time dinner reached us, and chocolate pudding tended to arrive with big lumps of unbeaten flour. When we had a visit from the dietitians at Middlemore Hospital, I took great delight in highlighting that the white bread they supplied for toast was a joke. It was all piled up for them to see at the back of the dining room where we had our meeting, so they couldn't avoid the question. They did make some changes after that, such as supplying wholemeal bread. However, my roommate and I decided to go halves in buying a loaf of Vogel's bread which lasted us a few weeks at a time. It was worth the extra expense!

The location of the spinal unit did have its upsides. A bakery, pizza outlet and Chinese takeaways were right next door. The fragrant smells wafting across our car park made it an easy and pleasant decision to venture over there some days, ditching Middlemore's wilted and soggy offerings in the process. By contrast, when the wind was in the right direction, we also had the distinct smell of hops from Dominion Breweries across the street!

Of course, friends sometimes visited with home-cooked

delights. Fifteen years later, I'm very conscious that food just ends up on the belly because I can't exercise it off. I can simply look at food and feel full, though food is still a comfort. I guess I just have it too good at home, being married to someone with a degree in cooking (technically, 'food science' but cooking sounds better.) That's why I married Jenny, after all!

One family I got to know at the spinal unit was the Remmerswaals. Lorraine Remmerswaal (now Mackie) comes from Rotorua, so we keep in touch and share a mutual understanding of what it's like to live with a spinal injury. Her son David was studying at the time, and the university allowed him to continue his studies while supporting his mum during rehab. Occasionally I had issues with my phone and David fixed it for me. Being younger, he was much more tech savvy than me. They are a lovely family, and David is one of those gentlemen who oozes a sense of grace and friendliness. He is now married with children of his own and runs a successful IT business. I've long since lost connection with the others who stayed in the ward with me, though we shared the joys and heartaches of the early months, adjusting to life with a spinal injury.

Each of us had regular physiotherapy and in some cases spent many hours getting set up for an electric wheelchair. Even though I'm right-handed, my left arm seemed to have more function after the accident because of nerve damage on my right. So they set up the wheelchair controls for me to operate on the left-hand armrest. I did get caught out on one occasion, driving into the steel support beam of the covered walkway between the gym and our accommodation. Of course, it happened right in front of the nurses' station, much to their delight!

In the end, I was determined to use my right arm. I reasoned that I already had 44 years of being right-handed, so it was more likely to function effectively in the long-term. Bear in mind that I'm in my wheelchair for approximately 12 hours a day on average, so it needs to work for me. We discovered that this approach was beneficial – I had just enough function to gain strength and build further coordination on the right. The joys of having tetraplegia (if one can say that) and triceps muscles that seize up with the cold mean that I need help with everything else.

There was a limited range of wheelchairs on offer at the time. I'm currently using a Swiss-made chair called a Levo. It's my third one and suits my daily needs. It has several electrically operated rams and actuators that coordinate to raise my wheelchair into a standing position. It means I can look someone in the eye when we're talking or preach in front of a crowd without a stage. It also has an electric tilt function which lets me rest different muscles, including my eyelids sometimes! I've clocked over 3,000 kilometres on average with each wheelchair. It mightn't seem much but in wheelchair terms it's a significant mileage when you consider all the costly componentry that's required to keep it functioning properly.

I have a second wheelchair which is more suited to the outdoors. It's called an Optimist and aptly named 'Optimist Prime'! When ACC first assesses you, they ask what your usual routines were before your accident. I made sure it was recorded that I accessed the Redwoods regularly for exercise and solitude. Had I not done that, I would have had to fight for another wheelchair, I'm sure.

Jenny and the boys would travel from Rotorua to see me at the weekends. By the time they arrived, I was usually in the dining room watching the TV news after dinner. I have vivid memories of Callum sneaking down the hallway and getting as close to me as possible without me seeing him. They stayed in one of three motel units which the spinal unit has for families of inpatients – I was going to say inmates!

Life with a spinal injury sometimes does feel like imprisonment, especially when I'm in bed in the evenings here at home, not able to reach over and give Jenny a back rub or get up speedily in the mornings. As an outpatient from the spinal unit, I have stayed there a few times over the years for various reasons when the motel units are available. They are a lot more accessible than other accommodation, which people often list as being wheelchair friendly but regularly is not! It's not uncommon for motels to have obstacles like lips on doorways, poky bathrooms, and limited space to store all my equipment.

On my first visit home to Rotorua from the spinal unit, the social worker organised for me to stay in a motel. I was determined to stay at home. He knew it but booked the motel anyway as per normal arrangements which are paid for by ACC. Our house hadn't been adapted for me at this point, but we made it work over the weekend. I remember pulling up in the driveway, thinking that this felt such a natural environment for me, yet aware that something incredibly different was going on in the way I exited the mobility vehicle and had to climb up the neighbour's driveway and into the house from around the back.

It felt natural and heartwarming to be in my own home environment with family and friends nearby. However, it was also a reminder that life was different now, underlining a reality that gave birth to a new dose of grief for me. Jenny and the boys made adjustments to our sleeping arrangements; poor Hamish had to exit his bedroom on the middle level and settle into a new space upstairs. Our master bedroom, also upstairs, became like a second lounge and gaming space for Callum.

Occasionally, when the family came to Auckland, we booked a van from the spinal unit and visited places around the city such as the beach, Sylvia Park Mall, and nearby parks. They made available an old Ford Transit and a Toyota Hiace, neither of which had good visibility for me, sitting in the back like a piece of roped-down furniture. These were precious times nonetheless – a chance to feel sea breezes and have an ice cream or fish and chips in public recreational spaces.

However, the weekends with my family ended all too quickly when Jenny and the boys had to drive back home to Rotorua, usually around 2pm on Sunday. I often wept as they took off in the Corolla. It was one of the toughest times for me while I was staying at the spinal unit. Little did I know that it would be even harder once I moved home permanently because the grief of losing so much function in my body hit me personally in the environment where I was so used to living independently, supporting family, helping friends and so on.

Mum and Dad were a tremendous help when they drove me back and forth for home visits from the spinal unit in Auckland. This meant driving from Tauranga in their own car and transferring to a rented mobility vehicle in which I could travel. After the trip, they made their way back to Tauranga. Dad says that it was an absolute privilege to help in this way, thinking nothing of the energy required to travel all those kilometres in a day. It relieved the pressure from Jenny who would otherwise make the journey with me.

On one occasion, I recall Mum sitting in the seat behind Dad, who was driving. She looked directly towards me. I was strapped to the floor in the back of the Toyota Hiace, as mentioned, like a piece of furniture. As we made our way across town, I started to cry. Rotorua is home. It just seemed so unfair and really tough to fathom. What was I doing heading back to Auckland? When I was a child, we often described Auckland as 'the big smoke'. As I was weeping, I noticed that mum was weeping with me too. Such was the nature of her empathetic heart. Words don't come close to describing how meaningful Mum's care was for me that day.

Empathy is a strong and powerful emotion, a gift that's close to my heart! (I'm holding back the tears as I record these moments on paper.) Mum and Dad have ached for me over the years, struggling to come to terms with the impact of my bike crash. The accident has taken a toll on the family, and I do not for one minute want to diminish the effect it's had on them.

On one planned visit home, I was asked to preach and take a baby dedication service at Rotorua Baptist. It was one of the children of our dear friends, the Edwards. On another occasion, a colleague named Fred Brunell asked me to preach at Mount Roskill Baptist in Auckland where he was senior pastor at the time. It was so fulfilling to continue with my craft of preaching despite my physical limitations. It's an incredible honour to open the Scriptures, to illustrate and share stories that encourage, challenge and motivate others on the journey of life and faith. Now, I had a fresh and evolving story to unpack, with all its complexities! This was the first of many opportunities that have opened up over the years.

There were about a dozen people staying at the spinal unit when I was there, ranging from a young 18-year-old to a woman in her 80s. They came from different walks of life: farmers, students, tradesmen and retirees, yet we were all going through the same struggles. It was not until some years later that I was able to understand more clearly about the grief that's associated with a significant traumatic event. As the Healthify website states about grief and loss, "Grief is the natural reaction to losing someone or something that you love or value."[6]

All of us need to identify grief and loss in order to understand and embrace it. That's been true for me. And, while grief is still triggered some days, I have hope, both in sharing daily life with awesome people from my community and in an eternal future from a Christian faith perspective. Significant relationships help and, I believe, are a sustaining factor for us all. Even brief and meaningful connections matter.

Occasionally, I was asked by the staff at the spinal unit to check in on one or two patients who had retreated into themselves and become overwhelmed by their plight. I felt so fulfilled in chatting with them and giving them hope, especially given that some folk in the ward had very few visitors. It helped heal my own pain and grief as well. I believe that each of us has unique experiences which equip us with the capacity to enhance and encourage others, regardless of our personality types. Despite my trauma, it was an incredible privilege to use my pastoral skills – to listen, weep, and occasionally pray for complete strangers, like family visitors who were struggling to get their heads around having their loved one go through this debilitating journey. If that's made a difference for them, then I'm fulfilled. Henri Nouwen was a Catholic priest, philosopher and author who devoted much of his life to helping people with mental health issues. He said,

> *Nobody escapes being wounded. We are all wounded people, whether physically, emotionally, mentally, or spiritually. The main question is not "How can we hide our wounds?" so we don't have to be embarrassed but "How can we put our woundedness in the service of others?" When our wounds*

cease to be a source of shame and become a source of healing, we can become wounded healers.[7]

Historically, inpatients used to stay for up to six months at the spinal unit. Once I had had three home visits, I reached the point where I was determined to get home in time for Christmas. After all, Rotorua was my home, not Auckland! Part of preparing to return home meant meeting regularly with the team of physicians involved in my rehab. They could see how determined I was, regardless of the progress I had made. The occupational therapist (OT) was the one to give the final okay and fortunately, she responded in my favour! On the day, I still required the neuro specialists to sign off my release. Need I mention that it took forever! Mum and Dad drove up, helped me pack, and brought me home, somewhat later than I'd hoped.

So, I made it home for Christmas, and recommenced pastoral work at RBC in March 2011. I was particularly enthusiastic about resuming my work amongst people I cared deeply about (picture 7). Despite the initial planning with the OT and social worker, several matters had to be addressed. We needed to organise support workers with the agency; establish new routines and sleeping patterns; acquire equipment like a memory foam mattress and a tilt table for physiotherapy; arrange a supply of consumables; get medication signed off from ACC; set up a temporary office downstairs in the church auditorium; arrange assistive technology support for computer and phone communication; and so on. The logistics were extensive. I was able to return to work gradually, starting with a few hours per day. Did I stick to that schedule? Not likely! And the social worker knew it! However, I did have the odd snooze in front of my computer or at least pretended to for a few weeks. And so, the next stage of my new life began, with all its nuances.

Questions for reflection:

What significant events have impacted your life in a traumatic or challenging way?

What have you learned from that experience?

How did the event impact your family, vocation, recreation, and spiritual journey?

How do you deal with grief and its ongoing impact?

How have you adapted to and found new significance in your journey?

What does it mean to be content while travelling a journey of grief?

What might you learn from travelling with me through my journey?

Chapter 3

People Really Do Care

As humans we are hardwired for relationships, for connection with others... In grief, as in so many aspects of our lives (and particularly times of traumatic and adverse events), our relationships with others are vital.
– Lucy Hone[1]

On the night of my bike accident, my family dropped tools and ran to be with me; fellow parishioners and friends came to my bedside; neighbours asked how they could help; colleagues spread the word; and local physicians tendered their skills on my behalf. I was surrounded by the best that humanity has to offer. Sadly, for whatever reason, the world is full of individuals who are destined to journey alone. I'm here to tell you that it shouldn't be that way. After all, even the Lone Ranger had Tonto!

Within each of us is the capacity to reach out and carry the hurting through uncertain territory, across rivers of despair, and onto hopeful shores. In small and large ways, I've been blessed with those who have reached out to care for my family and me. Firstly, let me illustrate this with the powerful and influential story of Job, as I've alluded to earlier.

Job's story is one of the earliest stories in the Bible. A farmer and well-regarded figure in ancient times, he was severely tested by Satan. In the space of weeks, he lost everything important to him: his family, his stock, most of his staff, and his health. The situation was so bad, even Job's wife suggested that he should curse God and die (Job 2:9). He had three friends called Eliphaz, Bildad and Zophar. They surmised that God caused Job's suffering because he'd committed some wrongdoing and deserved to be punished. This is the earliest record we have of this kind of thinking because Job predates the more well-known figure of Abraham.

It's not the focus of this book to unpack all the reasons why God allowed him to be tested by Satan. However, Job is relevant to my story, given his experience of suffering and survival. I don't believe it's in God's nature to harm us; nor does He actively wait for us to sin so He can punish us in response. Not discounting eternal judgement, I believe God is far too gracious to pursue us in such a disciplinary way, choosing instead to love all humans unconditionally, despite our shortcomings and misunderstanding of His ways.

In spite of their ill-conceived theological reflections, Job's mates did at least stand by him in his suffering, showing the true extent of their friendship toward him. In Job 2:11-13 we read that these friends heard of his adversity and travelled some distance to mourn with him and comfort him. On arrival they hardly recognised him.

Seeing his demise, they tore their clothes, threw dust over themselves and wept with him. Most of us are familiar with showing our support for others by having a cup of tea, spending a few hours consoling our friends, or those we encounter who may need some immediate pastoral support. Job's friends "...sat down with him on the ground for seven days and seven nights, and no one spoke a word to him, for they saw that his suffering was very great." (Job 2:13, NRSV) How about that for commitment!

In my opinion, this is one of the most powerful pictures of care and kindness. Contemporary Christian author Philip Yancey comments on the actions of Job's friends: "...I have learnt that simple availability is the most powerful force we can contribute to help calm the fears of others... Those were the most eloquent moments they spent with him."[2]

Dr Richard Tedeschi, professor of psychology at University of North Carolina, helped develop the concept of post-traumatic growth. He explores our coping mechanisms and acknowledges the place of others on the journey beyond trauma. In an interview with Lisa Bucksbaum, he was asked, "How can other people help?" He replied,

> *In some circumstances there really aren't words, sometimes it's just knowing that someone is there, and you can count on them. The expert companion is someone that stays connected to you. They don't have to be a medical practitioner, just someone who is prepared to stay with you for the long run.*[3]

The apostle Paul echoed this principle of care in the New Testament. To paraphrase 2 Corinthians 1:3-7 – God comforts us so that we can comfort others. And by doing so, we help them to endure their suffering. We are sometimes reticent or unsure how to help others in response to physical or psychological wounding, yet we recognise the importance of sharing that journey with them.

The late Dr Jared Noel and his wife Hannah decided to have a baby despite his terminal cancer. Family and friends managed to raise $170,000 in just a few days! This enabled them to purchase drugs to keep him alive long enough to see his daughter born and celebrate the first month of her life. With only six weeks to live, he documented his final reflections in the form of a book – *Message to My Girl*. He states, "It is impossible to find meaning in the context of suffering without a community of people around you."[4]

In essence, while recognising the different needs of extroverts and introverts, I believe we are creatures designed for communal living, not isolation, and certainly not to suffer in silence. We have four friends and acquaintances, each of whom have suffered with 'the big C' (cancer) since 2020. Each has chosen to share their journey with us, knowing that as close friends, we are on board with them: making meals, gardening, taking them to appointments, sending emails of support, listening, laughing, praying, weeping, and just being present with them. Each one receives a parcel of hope and strength as we share the journey, using whatever gift or resource we have.

I love Henri Nouwen's comments in this regard:

When we honestly ask ourselves which person in our lives means the most to us, we often find it is those who, instead of giving advice, solutions, or curses, have chosen rather to share our pain and touch our wounds with a warm and tender hand. The friend who can be silent with us in a moment of despair or confusion, who can stay with us in an hour of grief or bereavement, who can tolerate not knowing, not curing, not healing and face us with the reality of our powerlessness, that is a friend who cares.[5]

Technology has played a part in the care I've received. For example, when I was still in the spinal unit, Jenny gave me

Bluetooth earbuds. This gave me the freedom to call whomever I wanted, whenever I wanted. It also enabled others to connect with me. The staff at the spinal unit could be forgiven for wanting to remove that wretched device from my ear! "There it goes again; how am I supposed to do rehab with you when you're distracted by the phone all the time?" My earbuds were a vital channel of friendship and support in those early days, and they continue to play other important roles in my life, such as when I get stuck and need to call for help in the forest near home. Not that *that* happens much! Like all modern devices, they break down and wear out.

As previously mentioned, David Remmerswaal was my 'tech support'. David often came to my room and helped to solve problems when my phone or earbuds played up as I lacked the ability to diagnose the fault or push the appropriate buttons. He was a real gentleman who never seemed to flinch when I interrupted him.

Unbeknownst to me, another one of my friends and colleagues Rawiri (formerly Dave) Auty set up a Facebook page updating people with my progress after the accident. Rawiri had been my associate pastor at RBC, and we had become quite close, despite him moving to Taranaki a month before my accident. Rawiri's skills on the computer provided a forum where people from far and wide could journey with us and pray for us with relevant and specific information.

The whole church community rallied around, prayed for us and gave generously to support my family. Jason Mikaere was the RBC youth pastor at the time. He got together with Dave Moore, the pastor at the Apostolic Church at that time, and they set up a weekly prayer meeting on Sunday nights that was open to anyone. It's very humbling to recount this and to know that they sacrificed their time on our behalf. Like Rawiri, Jason, his late wife Horiana and their children (who were similar in age to our boys), had become very close.

I've since had the opportunity to preach and share my testimony with many of the parishes involved in that prayer meeting. It's been encouraging for them to see how God has responded to their prayers, and an important space for me to express gratitude for their support. In the same way, I've been invited to speak at most of the Baptist churches in the wider Bay of Plenty. My Baptist colleagues have been a tremendous backbone of support, not just for our family, but for many others who have experienced their own trauma.

I'm grateful to be part of a movement where reciprocal care is fostered. It's a reflection of our spirituality and the disciplines we embrace in the way we do church (our ecclesiology). Any of us can talk the talk, but can we walk the walk, that is, practise tangible expressions of love, kindness, generosity and gratitude? Surely, that's the essence of community.

For example, Jenny and I wanted to express our gratitude toward all those who helped and cared for me after my accident and in the ensuing days, such as ambulance, fire brigade, and hospital staff. Jenny made cakes and we even took one to ICU at Middlemore Hospital in Auckland!

Here is another example of being on the receiving end of care and support at a crucial time. On Sunday afternoon in the middle of March 2022 I developed a wheezy cough. I did a RAT (rapid antigen test) on Monday which showed a negative result for Covid-19, but the next day, I tested positive, most likely with the Omicron variant which had New Zealand firmly in its grip at that point. Jenny tested positive two days later.

I developed the common symptoms of a sore throat and

head cold, along with loss of taste and smell. I didn't have much energy, which compounded the fatigue that I battle most days. The hardest thing was getting rid of phlegm. I spent Tuesday in bed but got up on Wednesday and Thursday. Then on Friday morning, en route to the bathroom for a shower, I said to Bella, my support worker, "I don't feel well; my blood pressure is dropping." Moments later, I passed out.

Bella checked my pulse, which was fine, but she couldn't get me to respond. "You went pale and your eyes rolled back in their sockets," she told me later. Though nervous about leaving me alone for a minute, she rushed upstairs and woke Jenny who happened to be upstairs that night to get a little extra sleep. By the time they reached me, I was starting to wake up. Jenny asked me how I felt, but I was quite vague and unresponsive. So they took me back to bed, at which point I gradually improved!

I contracted Covid-19 again in the spring. However, that time I met the criteria to take antiviral medication, and it helped to take the edge off symptoms, despite the pills tasting horrible.

That first dose of Covid-19 left me with a wheezy cough, and the fatigue was quite prevalent two weeks later. The rest of our immediate family, apart from Callum, also came down with Covid-19 in winter that year. Many of our close friends dropped meals off at the front door, brought chocolate and sent messages of support while we were sick. We've been able to do the same for others since then. This kind of reciprocal care of each other speaks of community, and it pays lasting dividends, not only in our relationships, but also for our health and wellbeing. Robert Waldinger and Marc Schulz note:

> *If we accept the wisdom – and more recently the scientific evidence – that our relationships really are among our most*

valuable tools for sustaining health and happiness, then choosing to invest time and energy in them becomes vitally important. And an investment in our social fitness isn't only an investment in our lives as they are now, it is an investment that will affect everything about how we live in the future.[6]

As it happens, this fainting experience wasn't the first. About three months after my accident, my brother Steve visited me in the orthopaedic ward at Middlemore Hospital. The staff had seated me in a manual wheelchair and Steve started wheeling me down the corridor to get some fresh air in a different environment. Then, without warning, I fainted and passed out. He quickly wheeled me back to the room and helped the staff position me horizontally back on the bed. Though I didn't know it at the time, this episode was also due to an infection, this time affecting my bladder. Fainting and blood pressure issues are quite common for people with spinal cord injuries. I tend to barrel on with life and take them in my stride.

Another incident I recall was also from the early years after my accident. One of my support workers challenged me to try swimming. She cared for another client who did rehab exercises in the physiotherapist pool at one of the local retirement villages. How was this possible? I was reticent at first but decided to give it a go. It was quite a rigmarole. I needed two support workers for safety reasons. We had to bring my portable hoist in the van along with my sling and a change of clothes. I could book out the heated pool exclusively for $20, giving us approximately one and a half hours.

Once I was partly undressed, they hoisted me onto the water lift, spun me around and dropped me into the water. There was a range of buoyancy aids at hand. I was initially doubtful about the benefits of swimming, as I could barely move my arms and legs, but it was nice to be in the water, nonetheless. The best part was standing in the water near the edge of the pool. My support workers would grip my hands on the galvanised pipe in front, then push my knees until my legs locked in a vertical position, at which point, on a good day, I could remain standing in the buoyancy of the water for up to five minutes. It felt really good and gave my support workers a true impression of my height which is about 5 feet 10 inches or 178 centimetres.

The temperature of the swimming pool was around 35 degrees, almost spa pool warmth. It was kept at this level on purpose for the elderly folk there. It was a bit too hot for me, so occasionally I had the girls add some cold water. After nearly 45 minutes in the water, they lifted me back on to the lift as it was time I got out. Halfway up, I stated that I didn't feel too well. When they offered me a drink, I bit down on the bottle and passed out!

One of my support workers was a bloke called Tim Symington. He was tall and wiry, but very strong. I didn't know it until several minutes later, but he got behind me using the fireman's lift technique, and together with Jo Thompson, my other support worker, they lifted me out of the chair and placed me horizontally on the change table until I came to. The moment I lifted my head though I felt dizzy and struggled to respond normally.

The nursing staff just happened to be in training down the end of the hallway, a short distance from the physiotherapist rehab pool, so my support workers gained their attention. Two or three of them made their way briskly down to see if I was okay. They checked my vital signs which were within acceptable parameters. The trouble was, I couldn't lift my head very high off the mattress without feeling weak and unresponsive. So they rang the ambulance and off I went for a trip down to the hospital. Jenny met me there later in ED. Poor Jenny, I hoped she didn't feel too alarmed by this visit!

I had simply become dehydrated due to the heat of the pool, so they pumped me with fluids. We had organised for a few friends to come over to our place for dinner that evening; I managed to get home in time for dessert! I wasn't so keen on all the attention, but grateful to those who cared for me that day. The moral of the story was that I learnt to hydrate sufficiently before engaging in further rehab at the pool.

Some years later, at another pool session, I was about to exit the pool, and the water lift wouldn't work. The maintenance manager came and contacted a local plumber to remedy the fault. I remained in the water for some time, starting to shrivel up like a prune. My support workers Leuila Letoga and Debbie Matt gave me plenty to drink and cared for me. Eventually, the tradesmen repaired the water lift, and I was able to get out. I'm grateful to Leuila and Debbie who remained by my side, attending to my needs well past their allotted time to ensure that I got out of the pool, dressed and safely home.

Several months later, I was disappointed because the retirement village closed the pool to the public. I had enjoyed being there in the water and was sorry for the loss of this resource to the wider community as there were no other suitable facilities in Rotorua at that time.

Ironically, the recently opened $34 million QE Health Rotorua, which is New Zealand's only clinically integrated health and wellness centre, has two new rehab pools, but no suitable water lift for users like me to enter and exit the pool. Nor does it have suitable changing rooms. Nonetheless, the staff there are great, and we've negotiated to use the facilities with my own hoist and shower chair.

All my support workers sign up to address my daily personal needs. Supporting me through illness and meeting health and safety requirements are part and parcel of their job, but they have often gone above and beyond, as Leuila and Debbie did in the pool that day.

Another example was in August 2024 when I spent a night in hospital due to an infection in my big toe, which had begun to spread throughout my body, affecting my breathing and causing uncontrollable muscle spasms. There was a risk of sepsis, which can be triggered by blood poisoning from septicaemia.

Despite my reticence, Jenny contacted emergency services. My support worker Bella was on shift that night, so she accompanied Jenny and stayed with me to assist the ED staff with my care. Neither Jenny nor Bella had much sleep that night. It shows how much my support workers care and apply their craft with diligence. It means a lot to me.

Sometimes, I'm out on my own and need help from members of the public. One afternoon in the late summer of 2020, I told my support worker that I would wheel home from town. So she drove home and waited for me to turn up. My plan was twofold: firstly to have some solitude, and secondly to test my batteries as I'd been having trouble with them going flat. The curious engineer in me wanted to see what the story was! There are 10 indicator LED lights at the top of my control screen on the wheelchair – green, yellow and red. As the battery goes flat, each LED turns blue.

In town, I visited my cousin Pam Vincent's shop called Art United, which she ran at the time, to see her photo exhibition. I then rode a couple of streets over from Tūtānekai Street; just outside the Millennium Hotel I noticed that the first blue light had come up! So, instead of going any further, I decided to stay put and mitigate the risk of my batteries going flat at an inconvenient location between town and home. My next support worker was due to start in 20 minutes, so it made sense that she could pick me up instead of holding up the other one.

While I was waiting on the footpath, I met a parishioner from church who was just walking by to pick up her car after work. We chatted for about quarter of an hour, during which time a lake fly buzzed into my left ear. I said to her: "This is a bit of an odd request, but would you mind grabbing my sandwich wrap from lunch, which is tucked under my chest belt, and use it to remove the fly from my ear?" It was the nearest thing I could think of to alleviate my discomfort. "Of course, no problem!" she said. "What a relief," I thought. I didn't have to wait long before my next support worker arrived and took me home in the van. I had sufficient battery power to navigate our house until bedtime when my support worker placed my wheelchair on charge for the night, as per the usual routine.

I am intrigued by the number of times my need for help turns into the opportunity to help others. For example, one day, I was exploring a new track in the Redwoods near home. The new gravel was not yet compacted enough and I got stuck. Moments later a couple of guys stopped and pushed me onto a firmer part of the path. I continued, but it was clear that the path was getting worse, so I turned around, and immediately got stuck again! Anyway, who should turn up shortly after that but the same two guys. They were here on holiday from Holland, this time wielding a map and seeking help because they were lost. Once they got me unstuck again, I went with them and directed them back to the information centre.

On another occasion, I was cruising along and my wheelchair started slowing, becoming somewhat unstable at the same time.

I backed up and realised that I had accumulated a pile of leaves and twigs. Despite my best efforts, I came to a halt. Several people stopped to see if they could help; I recognised one as a local motelier. He was out jogging, pushing his two children in a double buggy. He explained that my rear wheel cluster had fallen off and the supporting axle had dug into the ground beneath me. I wasn't going anywhere at this point!

He asked the next jogger if he had come across my wheel. He hadn't, so the motelier and his two children turned around and headed back up the track to look for it. After some time, he returned, having found the wheel cluster and bolt shaft. That was great, I thought. However, he couldn't find the nut that held it all together. So, I got on the phone to our son Hamish who I knew would be just finishing work for the day. He said, "I'm on my way Dad." I was about 10 minutes away from the main car park nearby. He eventually turned up and supported me as I limped out of the forest on three wheels and made my way back to the van. What a relief to have his support that day!

In my experience, members of the public are generally more than willing to help if I grab their attention, rather than waiting for them to notice me. However, as I've experienced, some people can be far less virtuous at times. In July 2016, Jenny and I were visiting Auckland and stopped at Subway in the Manukau shopping mall for lunch. We were next in the queue waiting to place our order when a woman showed great disdain, walked straight by me to the front counter and began ordering her lunch. I couldn't believe her audacious behaviour. It was just as if I didn't exist. I could have taken offence and made a scene but chose to be silent on this occasion.

We underestimate the power of virtuous living, looking beyond offence, showing forgiveness and respect, going out of our way to show care and compassion to a stranger, or maybe even an enemy. Every day presents us with a choice to embrace opportunities and make a positive difference for others, no matter the individual or context. In a brief story from my daily devotional reading, Bob Gass recounted:

> *Prof Tony Campolo once attended the funeral of an acquaintance, and by mistake ended up at the wrong funeral parlour. The body of an elderly man was laid out, and his widow was the only mourner there. She seemed so lonely. Tony stayed for the funeral and then accompanied her to the cemetery. After the committal service, as they were driving away, Tony confessed that he hadn't actually known the lady's husband. "I thought so," she replied, "I didn't recognise you. But it doesn't matter. You'll never, ever know what this means to me."*[7]

I tend to just get on with life, and don't always see myself as having a spinal cord injury, even though it's physically obvious. I have to remember that my family carry on with life too, but not as they knew it. The impact for Jenny and the boys has been huge. Jenny has pressed on, responding to my daily needs, often putting herself second and being ever faithful to me. I love her to bits. It takes a fair amount to upset Jenny, though we sometimes experience tension and sadness together. I feel responsible for the impact my accident has had on our relationship and our family. We have had to work through the associated grief and loss, with particular focus on wellbeing and what that means for each of us.

Jenny's story

Responding to Tim's accident has meant adapting to a new normal – thinking about how to do life while juggling support for Tim under ACC, and Callum under the Ministry of Health (MOH). Each of them has very different needs. We had a handle generally on how to do life with Callum and autism. But now there is a tension with what's required to do the best for each of them. (And sometimes it is the opposite – Tim wants to be spontaneous and social, while Callum needs routine and predictability.) At the same time, we should not forget Hamish and his family's needs and how that plays out for all of us.

It was a steep learning curve with Tim in the beginning, as his life was so different before his accident – busy and active, enjoying our lovely Rotorua environment, biking, running, and kayaking. He and I lived interdependently then, but now he is totally dependent! We had to adapt and pivot, stepping in to do everything for him: giving him a drink of water, emptying his catheter, putting on his glasses, as well as doing the jobs he used to do around the house – mowing the lawn, house repairs, and vehicle maintenance. Then there was the shock of having support workers in the house most of the time. Spending those six months in hospital taught Tim a lot about how to live with tetraplegia, but there are things he would rather not have to face (as for all of us).

I can remember that ACC assessed him as having 92 percent loss of normal function. He can manage his wheelchair, but he can't feed himself, wipe his bottom or drive a vehicle. But we all need some help along the way, and it is okay to ask for help because there are always people who are willing to respond. Our journey is no different to yours in that respect, but people aren't mind readers, and everyone's needs are different. We've learnt the importance of telling others what is best for us and our whānau, with the realisation that life isn't static, that we all need to adapt and change.

Discovering this new normal has been a fluid journey. Sometimes it rushes by quickly and we barely have a minute to process what is happening around us. At other times, we are going slowly and feeling frustrated at the lack of progress. The analogy that I often use is that of a rollercoaster where, once you are strapped into a seat, you *have* to do the ride – you can't decide to get off halfway around. There are times on the ride when you are in the light and can see the track ahead, when you are able to anticipate where you are heading and prepare yourself. But other times, you are in the dark, getting thrown around as the carriage corkscrews down and around.

People often ask me how I live such a life. I guess I've been given a gift of faith in God, so I find it easy to trust God. To me, God is like the safety seat belt in the rollercoaster, holding me tightly and securely. Thus, I don't need to worry because He is dependable. In fact, my mantra is: "One day at a time." It sits on our dining table on a plaque, reminding me that between God, myself and our lovely community, I can do today! Tomorrow is so unpredictable and unknown; focusing on what is going to happen next month, next year, or next decade isn't helpful.

Adapting to a new normal raised some big questions for us as a family. Are we happy? What makes us smile? What brings us joy? Can a very broken man experience wellbeing? What about a young adult with autism? In terms of wellbeing, we have learned that it helps to have a positive approach to life. Tim and I conclude each day by focusing on what's been good. It directs our sense of gratitude and belief toward God; and the things that are truly meaningful contribute to our sense of wellbeing.

A good place to start answering these questions is by thinking about what matters to you, rather than what is the matter with you. This approach has been adopted by health professionals caring for the wellbeing of patients and families in Western Australia; as noted:

> *"What matters to you?" encourages more meaningful conversations between patients, carers, families and health care staff to help us care for patient's care is in line with their personal preferences and values. By asking, listening and responding to what matters to our patients, their families and carers, we promote person-centred care and improve outcomes.*[8]

This is a move away from negativity, which can all too easily grip us. According to the Oxford English Dictionary, the definition of wellbeing is 'the state of being happy, healthy or prosperous'. The rebellious side of me wants to disagree and challenge the dictionary, as it is not just about those three things; it is about how satisfied people are with their lives as a whole, involving their sense of purpose, their connection with others, and how in control they feel. Both Tim and Callum wrestle with what it means to be satisfied and purposeful, given their daily reality of brokenness in body and mind.

Jay and Katherine Wolf have written a book called *Suffer Strong: How to Survive Anything by Redefining Everything*. We have found this helpful in identifying the things that hold us back, though we are still able to have wellbeing and satisfaction at the end of the day.

None of us have unlimited access to whatever you want for whatever we plan for our lives to look like. We are constrained by our marriages or our singleness, by our children or our childlessness, by our obligations or our debts, by obstacles real or imagined. No one enters life or leaves it without feeling bound by something. Some of us have physical wheelchairs, but we all have invisible wheelchairs inside us. None of us can do life all by ourselves. We need God, and we need each other. Life with disabilities has been the most profoundly challenging and transformational experience of my life. It has given me a new perspective. It has invited me to lean into a different way of seeing God and living in the world. It has offered me a life of flourishing, not just in spite of my constraints, but because of them.[9]

This approach has been beneficial for us in terms of travelling the journey with others, caring for them, and being cared for ourselves.

We have learnt from two other models of wellbeing. The first is Te Whare Tapa Whā, a Māori model of wellbeing developed by Sir Mason Durie in 1984.[10] This model uses the analogy of a three-dimensional house, a holistic picture which considers the whole person and every part of their lives. It recognises that a stable house needs four walls to stand firm. The walls are taha wairua (spiritual wellbeing), taha hinengaro (mental and emotional wellbeing), taha tinana (physical wellbeing), and taha whānau (family and social wellbeing). These four walls are sitting on the whenua (land or roots), your place of belonging, where you feel comfortable and able to be you, whether at home, at work, at church, or at a friend's place.

Many other things can affect our wellbeing, apart from our

physical body, for example, if there is tension and stress in our family, or if we are struggling with global uncertainties such as pandemics, war or climate change. We may question whether God can be trusted to stand by us and care for us. Everyone's house or whare will look different depending on the things that impact their wellbeing.

The second model, Five Ways to Wellbeing, was adapted by the Mental Health Foundation from research done by the New Economics Foundation.[11] They outline five actions that, if built into everyday life, will help people gain a greater sense of wellbeing. Very briefly, they are:

1. **Connect** – Who is important to you? Who makes you feel valued? Who will stay in contact with you as a caring friend? It's important to maintain these connections and be realistic about our expectations of others; people are doing the best that they can with the best that they've got. I am blessed with my friends, my home group, my church and family. I love my grandma Fridays with Christopher, walking in the Redwoods and having a snuggle with our boisterous kittens.
2. **Give** – Sharing with others from what we have, whether it be time, words, a smile, or money encourages self-esteem and a sense of value and purpose. For me, giving away a bunch of homegrown flowers, taking a meal to someone, or being an advocate for a family living with autism are all actions that bring me joy.
3. **Take notice** – Paying attention to the present and what is happening, both inside and around us encourages us to relax in the busyness of life, to savour the moment, to be grateful and philanthropic. Dusk is my favourite time of day

when the dwindling light makes things look magnificent. I am so blessed to live on a hill from which I can see the failing light shining over the city every day. It's a beauty that reminds me of the creative hand of God in my life.
4. **Keep learning** – Being curious, setting goals, and trying something new are important for everyone. Callum and I try to visit the library weekly, and I love taking home books full of new learning and ideas. My family are also used to me with my air pods in, listening to a podcast while I am doing housework or gardening.
5. **Be active** – Moving your body is bound to make you feel better! Do whatever you enjoy, within your capabilities: bike riding, walking, swimming, or an exercise programme. It's even better if you can connect with others while doing it. My wristwatch has a step counter which vibrates to remind me to do 250 steps each hour.

It is difficult to focus on all these aspects at once; easier to just do one. I use an app that was developed after the Christchurch earthquakes. It's called 'All right?' You choose one of the five actions and receive a mini-mission every day. If you complete the mission, you get a reward and can then try another of the five actions. During the Covid-19 pandemic, I found it helpful to concentrate on the 'Connect' aspect. Now, a poster with all five actions is attached to my wall.[12]

I've reached the point now where I can say I am content with my life. It is hard to remember what life was like before Tim's accident, but we have learnt so many things and met so many amazing different people. We would have missed out on all that if it hadn't happened. I think that I am a better person for it. I have more empathy around disability, inclusion, grief and how these things affect whānau. I have more understanding – lived experience is definitely a teacher! And finally, I believe I have a broader relationship with God and others – focusing on love and wholeness. Who wouldn't want that!

Furthermore, contentment for me means being at ease or going with the flow. In other words, I wouldn't subscribe to feeling content 100 percent of the time, but mostly, it is recognising that life is just the way it is.

Honestly, we just need to live one day at a time as we don't know what is going to happen, especially when we are reliant on support workers. My friends smile when they ask how my week is going, and my reply is "Good!" if there have been no surprises! There are days when the phone rings at 6am and we have to scramble to fill that day's shift, trying to work out who in our team is available to support Tim (sometimes it's our friends or me!) Sometimes it means deciding which priority for the day is non-negotiable and what can be left. I can't change many of the circumstances of my life and generally people around me aren't trying to make my life harder. Some may recognise it as a cliché, but I think Reinhold Niebuhr's Serenity Prayer says it all:

God, give me grace to accept with serenity
the things that cannot be changed,
courage to change the things
which should be changed,
and the wisdom to distinguish
the one from the other.

Living one day at a time,
enjoying one moment at a time,

accepting hardship as a pathway to peace,
taking, as Jesus did,
this sinful world as it is,
not as I would have it,
trusting that You will make all things right,
I surrender to Your will,
so that I may be reasonably happy in this life,
and supremely happy with You forever in the next.

Tim's story

Several of our friends visited me at the spinal unit. Some of them were reticent, not knowing how to respond or what to expect when they saw me. Nevertheless, they came, and we talked about their lives and families as usual. I endeavour to make them feel relaxed, and try and act as normal as I can do under the circumstances.

On one weekend visit back to Rotorua, the church put on a dinner to welcome me home. It was an emotional time. I felt very self-conscious, wheeling into the church with all eyes on me. Many people had not seen me for months, yet they had prayed faithfully, fasted and interceded for us as a family.

The first person I noticed was a man I had supported pastorally over the years – Andy Valk. He was blind and had had a hard life, including a stint in prison, but he'd turned a corner by the time I got to know him in my first year at Rotorua Baptist Church. He was a larger-than-life figure who could play the drums and look after himself. Andy had a very cheeky laugh and an optimistic demeanour.

I made my way over to him and chatted with him and his wife Charlene. (I had had the privilege of marrying them a year earlier). I wanted to have more conversation time with them, but alas, there were plenty of other people to see. Andy and Charlene have both since passed away, each having had significant health issues. They had probably been living on borrowed time for many years.

Dinner was almost under way and a space was made for Jenny and me at the end of a table where several of our closest friends were seated. I used to pride myself on talking to as many people as possible at a party. On this occasion, I was comfortable to park at the dinner table and not have to canvass the whole room. What had changed? I guess I was grieving – feeling like a different person in a once-familiar environment. I found out later that our friends were protecting me from going home too tired after the event. I hugely appreciated the care, compassion and hospitality shown to us by everyone that night.

The next morning at church, I was asked to preach and take a child dedication for our good friends Phil and Amy Edwards. My mate Keith Turner didn't expect that I would do both, but you couldn't hold me back. This was my church, and I was amongst friends; I saw it as an opportunity to serve with the gifts God had given me. Jenny ably supported me on stage, helping with my notes, and some of the props for the children's dedication. Another friend, Alma Emery, commented to my wife and several others afterwards: "Tim's just the same!"

The good folk at Rotorua Baptist Church have helped us in many practical ways over the years. In particular, friends Terry Schick, Chris Thompson, and Ian Jackson chopped down trees, and split, delivered and stacked firewood for us until we retrofitted a gas boiler to power the central heating. It's a convenient reminder of how blessed we've been by the friends and associates who helped to keep the wood boiler running for years. It was always very hungry for wood! Others have helped with gardening, house decorating, maintenance jobs, tidying my garage and workshop, shifting furniture, tightening door hinges or simply securing screws that may have come loose on a window latch or piece of furniture.

As a practical person myself, I'm extra grateful to friends and neighbours who have offered their practical skills at home. Ray Hewlett comes over from next door to mow our lawns, meticulously doing the edges and using a leaf blower to tidy up the mess when he's finished. He has become part of my story and blesses us as a family. All those who live in Janet Place mean such a lot to us here in the Lee household.

Initially, before our house modifications in 2012, the only way to get into the house was up our neighbour's driveway, around the back of our house and into the lounge via our internal deck. Even this would not have been possible without Ian Jackson and Bob Fitzsimmons who chopped down a tree and laid a concrete pathway connecting the neighbour's driveway to our back deck.

There were some people whose help I didn't find out about until later; people like Philippa Lewis (née Pedersen) who owns a commercial laundry business and did laundry for Jenny and the boys for some time. I feel so humble that she blessed us in that way. Neighbours Pete and Penny Ricard graciously allowed me access off their driveway. Pete even fabricated a steel ramp, which enabled me to wheel over the concrete kerb. ACC usually covers the cost of such modifications, provided they've accepted a quote beforehand. In this case, my mates simply got stuck in and made it happen so that I could access our living areas as soon as possible on returning home. Fortunately, we were able to retrieve the cost of concrete and materials from ACC after the event – not without some discussion though!

Some friends blessed us by thinking of basic needs, like

warmth in the winter. Close family friend Adalene Taylor has knitted me several winter scarves from angora goats' wool, two of which remain tied to my wheelchair. I use them regularly each winter. She also knitted me a small blanket which remains in our dining room and gives added warmth for my legs on the days when we don't have our central heating on. Adalene is an example of someone thinking about practical needs that we might otherwise take for granted. She has been like a second mum to me over the years and goes the extra mile to use her skills in a loving and caring way.

My mates have been there to support me in different ways over the years. Whilst I'm not a fan of Auckland traffic, the city's proximity to the ocean is a redeeming factor. I've discovered that I can head east towards Howick, park the van at the Half Moon Bay marina and catch the ferry into the central city and the Viaduct Harbour. It saves a lot of hassle trying to find a park in lower Queen Street. And it means I get to enjoy a boat ride, the smell of sea air, and the views of Auckland's clifftop mansions on the way. I love the ocean. In the past, Jenny and I went on several sailing adventures to places like Kawau Island and Great Barrier Island.

I've probably made this trip about half a dozen times now. It makes for a long day after leaving Rotorua around 7am and returning about 12 hours later, but it's well worth the effort. Chris Thompson was the first to drive me from Rotorua to the marina where I met up with friend Paul Collins who lives nearby in the suburb of Dannemora, Botany. Paul and I spent time looking at the super yachts and eating fresh fish and chips from the fish market.

My dad and brother Steve have also driven me there and we've enjoyed quality time together beside the ocean. Steve had to drive from his home in Hamilton then, sometimes staying the night with us on return to Rotorua from Auckland. Steve is a competent sailor, so we enjoyed visiting the Viaduct Harbour when Auckland hosted the America's Cup in March 2021. We had plenty to talk about in relation to boats!

In thinking about caring for others in their moments of struggle and trauma, I've been inspired by the story of Kiwi Nikki Hamblin and American Abbey D'Agostino who competed in the 5,000-metre heat at the Rio Olympics in August 2016. Hamblin stumbled and fell down on the track. D'Agostino, running closely behind her, then tumbled over her and landed badly. Hamblin stood and helped D'Agostino to her feet, then continued running briefly. She looked behind to see that D'Agostino had started running again but was clearly badly injured and fell a second time. Hamblin turned back and encouraged D'Agostino to keep running. So, D'Agostino finished the race in pain and was taken off the track in a wheelchair with a torn ligament in her knee (ACL). Despite not qualifying in their heat, they were both given permission to compete in the final, although D'Agostino was too injured to compete any further. Each received the Pierre de Coubertin Medal for demonstrating the spirit of Olympics.

I love the character shown in both these competitors. D'Agostino said, "By far the best part of my experience of the Olympics has been the community it creates, what the games symbolises. . . Since the night of the opening ceremonies, I have been so touched by this – people from all corners of globe, embracing their unique cultures, yet all uniting under one celebration of the human body, mind, and spirit,"[13] while Hamblin commented, "My result on the track doesn't define who I am as a person."[14]

I think it's a wonderful picture of two people sharing a tough journey in a moment of suffering, even though Hamblin gave up the possibility of winning a medal after years of training in her specialist event. As Mother Teresa famously said, "God does not require that we be successful, only that we be faithful."[15]

The world would be a different place if we all showed the kind of care and sacrifice that Hamblin exhibited that day.

> *Now we who are strong ought to bear the weaknesses of those without strength, and not just please ourselves.* (Romans 15:1, NASB)

Our close friends are still on the journey with us. I am eternally grateful and humbled by the care and attention I've received. We take every opportunity to reciprocate their support, and long may it be an example to those looking on.

> *Bear one another's burdens, and thereby fulfil the law of Christ.* (Galatians 6:2, NASB)

Questions for reflection:

Who are the most significant individuals in your journey of life, and why?

What are the qualities of a good friend?

How has the way people treated you influenced the way you treat others?

What are the implications of journeying alone while trying to maintain your wellbeing?

List the most helpful ways that people have supported you. Take time to express your gratitude to them.

How does the relationship between Job and his friends influence your friendship with others?

How have the wellbeing models that Jenny mentioned been most helpful to you?

Chapter 4

Getting the Right Help

...What you have to learn to accept when you're disabled, is that our ability to control the care that we receive, that interdependence we have with support workers and with providers. That is what independence looks like. That is what freedom looks like in this body...
– Amanda Lowry[1]

How does general day-to-day life work for a bloke in my position? I'm completely reliant on the help of others to get me up each day, to live independently and remain mobile wherever my vocational, social and recreational needs take me. Accident Compensation Corporation (ACC) funds all my personal needs, equipment, transportation and house modifications as necessary.

ACC was established and legislated in 1972 as the result of A Royal Commission of Inquiry into compensation for injury in 1966. In my opinion, we are really blessed to have this service in Aotearoa New Zealand, a service that in 2023/24 cost ACC about $2.04 billion in new claims, benefiting almost one-third of New Zealanders (according to ACC statistics).[2]

The ACC process for compensation begins with a serious injury needs assessment. The higher the level of injury, the greater degree of support needed. In my case, this was done first at the spinal unit and is reviewed through further assessment every two to three years, with decreasing regularity as the years go by. The reason for this is because functional ability may change, often improving in the first couple of years in the case of an incomplete spinal injury like mine. Other factors like vocational and recreational pursuits influence the outcome of assessments and the level of support that ACC contributes. I was told that after two years, whatever level of ability you have is generally what you are stuck with. That's been generally true for me.

The assessment process allocates support depending on my daily needs. ACC funds almost 24/7 care for me (around 148.5 hours per week). On returning home from the spinal unit, individual clients are assigned a caseworker to manage their support contract. ACC had a local office here in Rotorua back in 2010, so we had personal face-to-face interaction with support staff there. Through a variety of reforms, structural changes, and cost-cutting exercises, ACC decided to centralise their systems in 2020, sadly disbanding the case managers at our local office in the process.

Since that time, I've mostly interacted with case managers from out of town. Ironically, more recently, they have reinstated case managers at the local office! Generally, I've had great support from these case managers, though my first one was not very personable, making it hard work at every turn. I've learnt to be thick-skinned and proactive in this business.

Many clients are not aware of their entitlements and thus don't always receive the care and support they need. It took some time for us to know the right questions to ask and the right language to use. Having the right advocates is essential when keeping ACC accountable too, because they don't always get it right!

Towards the end of 2017 a debate arose with my case manager about the times when Jenny should be paid to support me. She wasn't getting paid to support me at my speaking engagements because this was regarded as 'natural support', and therefore did not comply with ACC's obligated compensation for 'attentive hours'.

Jenny raised the issue with the case manager who agreed that some payment was fair enough, but that I should have a new needs assessment done. In April 2018, an assessor came to our home and went through the usual questioning of what I do every minute of every hour of every day. It's understandable that ACC have parameters to work within, but it feels very degrading and intrusive as a client, let me tell you! The assessment report came through, and we were horrified to be told by the case manager that, "Timothy could have his attendant hours reduced as he is only doing volunteer work instead of paid work."

In fact, I've been doing a mix of paid and unpaid work since the beginning of 2016, and my compensation is abated on declaration of income. That means every time I declare income, they reduce what they pay me by an amount close to that. That in itself is discouraging from a financial perspective. You can understand why some people with spinal injuries don't bother with paid work at all! We felt that the needs assessor had not understood my needs sufficiently, that I was being unfairly penalised, and that Jenny's support was misrepresented even though she is my wife.

We educate people that Jenny is firstly my wife, secondly my personal assistant, and thirdly my support worker at times. So, we disputed the assessment. Five months later, in September, we were told that a reduction of maybe six or seven hours per week was likely. The whole situation became quite stressful for me, as I was doing my best to fulfil an interim pastorate at St John's Presbyterian at the time. I was feeling down and withdrawn and Jenny conveyed to my ACC case manager that my mental health was affected. She referred them to the Mental Health Foundation of New Zealand's best practice guide:

> The Mental Health Foundation believes one of the key aims of a democratic government is to promote the good life: a flourishing society where citizens are happy, healthy, capable and engaged. In other words, a society where people have high levels of wellbeing. Recent years have seen a shift away from a focus on illness alone, to more attention on wellness, both in policy and health practice... Illness and wellness are now considered to be more than simply two ends of a continuum, but separately operating dimensions.[3]

I've done my best to create a meaningful life after losing so much, and I shouldn't be hindered from making it work for me. After all, I love serving the people of our community and beyond. It's a meaningful pathway and contributes to my sense of wellbeing. As the Mental Health Foundation's brochure states: "The wellbeing of individuals is bound up in the wellbeing of their communities."[4]

Despite agreeing that it was not conducive to my wellbeing, they sent a letter in October stating that 20 *hours* would be removed from my care package, potentially commencing in November. We felt bullied, and that our right of reply was nullified. After extensive communication, our case manager suggested that it might be best to have another needs assessment done, to which we agreed. Despite this, ACC informed us at 5pm on the last working day of the year just before Christmas that my care package would be reduced by 20 hours in January!

We felt very much isolated and helpless at this point. I decided to reach out to my Baptist colleagues in case they knew of anybody who could help us. My colleague Ross Banbury, who was pastoring at Te Puke Baptist, had a good friend who was a lawyer. This man had spent much of his legal career working in the commercial sector but saw some of the injustices for recipients of accident compensation. He focused his energies in this direction out of a compulsion to help. We contacted him and learnt that he acted for most ACC case reviews in the country at that time. This gave us some hope, so we engaged his services. He set to advocating on our behalf.

When a notice of review is sent to ACC, they usually request a conciliation process as a way forward; this is not surprising, because case reviews become public documents! So, on 22 August 2019, Jenny, the lawyer and I had a meeting with the case manager and an experienced conciliator to present our case. Despite our beef with ACC, we had a good relationship with my case manager and were surprised that she turned up to such an important meeting on her own.

We had prepared extensively and argued that my ability to work, whether voluntary or paid, would be impeded if their decision was upheld; that Jenny deserved to be recognised fairly within my care package; and that I should be the best person to decide how my care is implemented. To cut a long story short, after what became a year of heartache, we won the case and it cost ACC a lot of money to pay us out, including recompense for the lawyers' expenses. Our tax on the settlement was quite significant though!

The next ACC needs assessment resulted in reinstatement of a full and comprehensive care package that met my needs and acknowledged Jenny's support. We've never had a problem with ACC since that time! In fact, they've been more than accommodating of my needs, and we continue to be grateful for their support.

In spite of some struggles, I am blessed to have the help of ACC and continue to work hard at reflecting what's truthful and fair in relation to the help they provide. I support the fact that ACC is not a free-for-all claims funding organisation, and it's unfortunate that people abuse the system sometimes. However, I'm seeking to use their funding with integrity to meet my needs.

A significant amount of ACC funding goes toward my support workers, through the agency HealthCare New Zealand. I have a team of six or seven support workers generally. Most of them are immigrants, along with one or two local Kiwis, depending on their career studies or gap year interests. I've had different ones from India, Fiji and Canada in the past, but a mix from the Philippines and Samoa is generally the makeup of my support team now. Up until recently I've only had one New Zealander on the team at any given time.

One recent example was Haidee. She started work with me in July 2022 during the first year of her nursing training. She is young, teachable, a fast learner, and was pleasant company to have in our home. I've had a few nursing students like her over the years. They have proved to be very successful, often procured through word-of-mouth amongst our circle of friends and colleagues. Haidee is the daughter of a lovely lady who worked as a staff administrator at St John's Presbyterian where I was an interim pastor for a few years (picture 17), and where I currently work as a part-time chaplain to one of their community-facing ministries. Sadly, as with other nursing students, I lost Haidee when she resigned to take up a full-time position as a registered nurse in 2025.

It was very difficult finding support workers during the Covid years, due to factors such as fewer immigrants coming into the country, vaccination mandates, and sickness affecting the healthcare industry at large. I read one story from July 2022 about a 71-year-old Tauranga resident who had paraplegia. Her support worker called in sick, but nobody provided cover for her. The client was left alone in a wet and bloodied bed for three hours.[5] Three years on, HealthCare New Zealand continues to face a shortage of disability support workers.

By contrast, I've been blessed with a wonderful support team who have served me faithfully and reliably over the years. They attend to all my personal and rehab needs, ranging from passive exercises to getting me up each morning – toileting, showering and dressing. Furthermore, they are there to support my daytime work-related routines, recreational activities, driving to appointments, speaking engagements, and voluntary community service. They also help with daily household chores, staying overnight (usually four nights per week), administering medications, and so on. I pretty much need help with everything, apart from driving my wheelchair. And I even need help with that on a bad day when the weather is cold outside, and my muscles seize up! The cold also causes my muscles to spasm uncontrollably when I hit slight bumps. This makes it hard navigating doorways and uneven road surfaces.

The more experienced support workers can drive the wheelchair inside from the laundry of our house where it's charged overnight, down the narrow hallway and into our bedroom ready for me. They are usually very reluctant to try this at first, as with driving our Mercedes Sprinter van. I encourage them as much as possible to give things a go. I'm a fan of bringing out the best in people and giving them confidence to tackle a wider range of tasks. As time goes on, I can see from their body language that they are quite proud of what they've achieved, especially when it comes to driving a larger vehicle than their own car.

My support workers become part of the family, and we seek to advocate for them as much as possible because they are generally loyal and supportive, covering extra shifts when others are sick or on leave, for instance. As another client's support worker said, "You become quite committed to the people you work with when you've been working with them long-term. You pick up extra shifts to help and you don't want to see them go without."[6]

I have no hesitation in contacting HealthCare New Zealand's People and Culture department on my support workers' behalf. I have to go through a facilitator as a primary means of communication now. Previously, I was part of a client advisory group which included agency reps including HR, relationship managers and service facilitators. We met alternately in Hamilton or Rotorua.

Jenny and I work hard to accommodate my support workers' holiday breaks. Mostly we organise cover from within the team, though occasionally we use on-call workers from the agency. I avoid that as much as possible because it takes significant time and energy just to get up in the morning, let alone working with strangers who aren't familiar with my routines. It's not just the up-close and personal nature of the job but having to talk them through everything that needs to be done during the shifts. I've had people turning up smelling of cigarette smoke or dressed inappropriately; it's not pleasant. Sometimes when on holiday, I just can't avoid that. As much as I can explain my needs to the agency, they might send support workers with little experience, particularly if they are struggling to find staff.

On one such occasion in Wellington, we were spending Christmas with Jenny's family. A young lass came to help me with the morning routine. After giving me a shower and getting me dressed, she hoisted me into the wheelchair with Jenny assisting from behind. I was almost fully in when I must have accidentally knocked the auxiliary power button in my headrest. The support worker leaned on my joystick which propelled the wheelchair backwards and pinned Jenny up against the French doors behind her. The support worker then pulled the joystick the other way, unaware how sensitive it is. Unfortunately, it propelled the front of my wheelchair up her leg and knocked her onto the couch beside us. She went home limping and never turned up the next morning! Jenny was relieved that the wheelchair hadn't smashed the glass in the French door, especially since it was Christmas Eve. Fortunately, she came out unscathed, unlike some other times when assisting holiday support workers.

On another occasion we were on holiday at Ōhope Beach and there were no support workers available to help me. The agency tried extensively to procure somebody local, but to no avail. So they organised a man to drive over from Hamilton to help me. We got a call from him partway to say that his vehicle had broken down on the main road near Pukehina Beach. So Jenny secured me in the van and we drove to pick him up from the side of the road. His dad had to drive over, pick him up and retrieve his vehicle on a trailer a few days later.

Jenny is incredibly faithful and supportive to me, acting as my PA, administrating the rosters for my support workers, and communicating necessary information to ACC when we go on holiday. She picks up the pieces when our property gets damaged, takes me to appointments, and covers for some shifts when a support worker is sick. I desperately wish I could swap places with her, not wishing the injury on her, but to be the one serving her, expending time and energy, and making sacrifices on her behalf. This is an ongoing tension for me to live with. As fellow Kiwi Amanda Lowry, who also lives with tetraplegia, aptly said, "I don't always want to be just another job for my family to do."[7]

Jenny and I have intentionally put boundaries around some of the personal care she does for me. She is my wife after all, and we want to guard that relationship for the sake of our marriage. It's a personal decision which other families in our situation choose to adapt in varying ways. In the story I mentioned earlier, the Tauranga resident "...said her husband was the 'unpaid helper' but did not want to be a caregiver. He refuses because we're entitled to care through ACC, and it's very hard in your marriage, having somebody to do their care."[8]

Neurosurgeons Timothy Beutler and Lawrence Chin noted in 2024:

> *The divorce rate annually among individuals with spinal cord injury within the first 3 years following injury is approximately 2.5 times that of the general population, whereas the rate of marriages contracted after the injury is about 1.7 times that of the general population.*[9]

These statistics are quite sobering. On the other hand, they appear to show that people are still willing to sign up to a long-term relationship, fully knowing what that might involve. It shows the level of care and compassion that some people are willing to extend toward a loved one with a spinal cord injury. We know such a person whose support worker became his wife. To this day they remain in a committed and loyal relationship. I'm so grateful to Jenny for standing beside me through the thick and thin of life as it is now. We have our tough days like any couple. The added dimensions of my disability, a son with unique needs, ongoing interaction with ACC, support workers coming and going every day, and so on, mean we rely a lot on the grace of God and the care of friends and family simply to survive. It's no wonder God only gives us 24 hours at a time to worry about!

I call on the boys to help me occasionally. Our son Hamish is very intuitive when assisting me in situations like this; he knows just what I need without me having to explain the solution to a problem. Before our house modifications were carried out and when Hamish still lived at home, I had to exit at the middle storey of our house to access the neighbour's driveway. It's a relatively steep slope which can get slippery with moss in places. Sometimes my arm would seize up during the cold winter months as I navigated my way down toward the road. Hamish would sometimes take over and drive the wheelchair down, along the footpath and back up our driveway to the shelter of the van in front of our garage. I feel confident in his ability to help me reach the places I need to go.

Like Hamish, Callum is incredibly caring and comes out with me on Thursday afternoons for our weekly father-and-son time. We go to the movies, up the gondola, visit the shops or have an ice cream by one of our local lakes or parks. This remains a precious weekly time to share together. During this time, while my daytime support worker goes off to do an errand for me or have their break at a local coffee shop, Callum will attend to my immediate needs effectively. He has a very caring heart and feels that it gives him real purpose, looking out for his 'old man'! I'm grateful for this, though I wish I didn't have to call on family to help at all. I figure they deserve not to be burdened by their husband and father.

As far as ACC's legal obligations are concerned, Jenny does get paid as part of my support team, as do our two boys. They are classified as 'natural support', which means there are times when they are paid in a limited capacity, or not at all, simply because they are immediate family. This is fair enough in principle when they're living under the same roof and available to help at times. However, the system falls short if ACC assumes family are available on tap!

There was a time when family members were not recompensed for their efforts at all. In a landmark case, which commenced in 2005 and went before the Human Rights Review Tribunal (HRRT) in 2008, the wife of Mr Atkinson argued that she should be paid as a carer because she wanted to help her spouse. Atkinson's injury happened pre-ACC, when the Ministry of Health (MOH) was the predominant funder of specialist health care. In 2015 Rosemary McDonald gave her perspective on the findings of the Tribunal, writing:

> *Coming from what we suspect was a position of almost complete ignorance, the Tribunal members were forced to go to a disability 101 default setting... The Tribunal grasped the inadequacies of the Needs Assessment and Service*

> Coordination (NASC) process, and they examined in some depth the utterly nonsensical concept of 'natural supports,' on which the NASC system is predicated.[10]

In her article, McDonald cited the Ministry of Health (MOH), Department of Social Services (DSS) and ACC joint service specification for home and community support services which stated that: "It would seem artificial to us to make a distinction as to payment options to family members for home care, purely on the basis of the cause of the disability."[11] It's ironic that ACC clients are currently far better served in terms of funding and services compared with MOH clients, who've been administering the NASC process.

I regularly meet people who deserve far better funding and services than they get under MOH. They may have non-accident-related medical conditions, such as cancer, multiple sclerosis or a stroke. This inequity means that some people with limited means are unable to afford necessities, like wheelchairs.

Furthermore, there is ongoing uncertainty around the support that MOH clients receive, despite their genuine needs, as is the case for our son, who comes under the NASC system. As a result of cost pressures felt by Whaikaha, Ministry of Disabled People, the current Minister for Disability Issues, Hon Louise Upton, commissioned an independent review of the Disability Support System (DSS) in September 2024. The upshot of this, according to Whaikaha, is that NASC will now be administrated by the Ministry of Social Development (MSD). "Disability Support Services (DSS) and related functions were transferred from Whaikaha to MSD, as a branded business unit, from mid-September 2024."[12]

In terms of my personal care support, ACC has funded my van, modifications to our home, my wheelchairs and the ongoing maintenance required to keep them going, plus hundreds of thousands of dollars in medical care and sundry supplies. According to my calculations, ACC spent between $450,000 and $500,000 every year in the first 10 years after my accident!

ACC Minister Matt Doocey announced an independent review of ACC in December 2024, out of concerns for the declining rehabilitation rates and increasing costs. In my experience, ACC has always expressed a desire for its recipients to be rehabilitated, independent, and in some kind of work. Despite my current mix of paid and unpaid work, I feel somewhat heartened by his comments, "I know that many Kiwis are doing it tough. The staging of the increase in ACC levies reflects this."[13]

It's important to my independence that we can have holidays away, in spite of the logistical challenges. Sometimes we take my own support worker and sometimes we have been able to obtain local care. In 2014, we booked a family trip to the Gold Coast for two weeks. It took about eight months of planning! Everyone told us we would have to take my own support worker with us and pay for their associated accommodation and travel expenses. However, I managed to locate a Gold Coast agency called Just Better Care who supplied a support worker for me for the time we were there. It worked out very successfully. We organised a private contract with them and ACC paid Jenny for the full time we were away. The difference in what we paid was minimal, so that helped mitigate the expenses for our trip.

I also located a specialist wheelchair technician in case my wheelchair broke down. Fortunately, that didn't happen! I took my wheelchair, shower chair, portable hoist, all the chargers and associated equipment which I would normally take when we go away on holiday in New Zealand. Air New Zealand was very helpful. We learnt that one of their pilots had a son with a spinal injury and travelled regularly with him.

We were also grateful to a friend, Bob Symon, who gifted us a week's free accommodation during our two-week stay at a timeshare resort in Coolangatta. Bob is the son of Ann Clausen, a lovely lady at Rotorua Baptist Church, and has a high-level spinal injury similar to mine. What better person to recommend a place to stay!

Our adventure to Aussie began with Jenny, the boys and me travelling to Auckland from Rotorua the night before. They all helped get me into bed and up in time for an early trip to the airport the next morning. I slept in my clothes, and we got going at 3am in order to check in on time. No shower that day! After exiting the departure lounge, I wheeled onto the rear tailgate of a small truck/bus and was hydraulically lifted to gain level access inside. There was a handful of us who required extra assistance boarding the plane, so we were first to board. The truck made its way out onto the tarmac and backed up to the front entrance of the aircraft. Up we went with the help of the truck's hydraulic scissor-lift until just short of the height for level entry to the plane. Oh dear; it wouldn't go all the way! After several attempts, they called for a technician to solve the problem.

As we waited, Callum became anxious about the delay, and he could see a bus on the tarmac with the bulk of passengers waiting to board the plane after us. At that moment, Hamish noticed that my trouser leg was wet. Jenny had no choice but to undo my trousers in front of others to investigate and discovered that the tube of my catheter which ran down my leg had become disconnected. Other than reconnecting my catheter tube, there was no other solution to the problem of wet pants. I would have had to get out of the wheelchair, onto a bed, change into clean trousers, then reverse the entire process! Eventually they fixed the scissor-lift, we boarded the plane, and I travelled to Australia with wet trousers!

The airline had a special hoist called an 'eagle lifter' which lifted me out of my wheelchair and was used to wheel me down the narrow aisle of the plane to our seat. It still required some manhandling by Jenny and two of the air hostesses. On arrival at the Gold Coast, they had a similar hoist and hydraulically operated platform which retrieved me from the plane. The staff unpacked my wheelchair and equipment from the hold of the plane and met us on the tarmac. Then, Jenny and Hamish used my hoist to put me back into my wheelchair. At last, I had a modicum of control over my life! At that point, airport staff gave us priority access through customs, and we made our way past the long line of passengers out to the car park where I had arranged a rental company to meet us with our specially adapted Volkswagen Caddy, our transport for the two weeks on the Gold Coast.

We enjoyed staying at the resort in Coolangatta. It was right on the beach with a wide concrete path in front of the sand dunes that accessed a range of beaches on the peninsula. Locals informed us that the sea breezes meant it was a more comfortable place to stay than further north in central Gold Coast. We discovered that it was five to ten degrees cooler than just 15 minutes' drive up the road! We settled into the hotel and went for a drive to get our bearings. We pulled over at a park next to the tidal river that accessed Tweed Heads. For a tidal river, it was stunningly clear water, unlike what you'd see in New Zealand.

I was anxious to explore further and could see some high-rise hotels not far in the distance. So I told Jenny and the boys that I would meet them there in about half an hour. It didn't look far away, so I took off on my own. Having reached the hotels, I waited for some time. It was clear that I should have been more specific. Essentially, we lost each other due to my vague directions. Ooops!

I had to ask someone on the beach if they could ring Jenny to direct them to my location because we hadn't paid for roaming in Australia. It was beyond dinner time when they eventually caught up with me. I wasn't very popular with my tired, stressed and hungry family! Little did we realise that in fact I was at Rainbow Point, the beach next to Coolangatta, just a few streets away from our hotel!

In the time we were staying there I made my way around the area quite comfortably, enjoying precious times of solitude by the ocean. One day we organised a trip to the movies in central Coolangatta nearby. By the time we arrived at the theatre, we were confused as the movie was halfway through. We looked at our phones which showed the time was an hour later! It turns out we had crossed the border between Queensland and New South Wales which goes right through the middle of Coolangatta. That one-hour time difference had thrown us! Alas, seeing that movie had to wait until sometime later back home in New Zealand.

As a treat for Hamish, I arranged a drive in a V8 supercar at a track further south from us – not a bad activity for a petrolhead! Callum enjoyed the hotel swimming pool and shopping for surprises. We travelled around the Gold Coast, visited nearby Currumbin Wildlife Sanctuary, shopped at IKEA, took a lift up the tallest hotel in Australasia, and enjoyed catching up with some friends from New Zealand.

Our close friend Amanda Turner was living at Southport at the time. She had recently moved from Rotorua and had formerly attended the Baptist Church when I was the senior pastor. We made our way north from Coolangatta to visit her and arrived in time to join the service at her church. As we made our way into the auditorium, the pastor greeted us and reached forward to shake Hamish's hand, assuming that he must be the pastor from New Zealand. Was it Hamish's good looks, or the fact that I was in a wheelchair that led him to believe I couldn't have been the pastor? Alas, it wasn't the first time I was on the receiving end of such assumptions!

After enjoying a barbecue together, Hamish noted that our rental vehicle was showing 38.5 degrees as we drove south back to our resort. Boy it was hot!

Chris and Lauren Downs plus their two children also drove down from Brisbane to visit us one day. We had become good friends with them when staying in Levin during the late 1990s and early 2000s. Lauren taught with Jenny at Waiopehu College, and they attended the Baptist church with us at that time.

Jenny and the boys faithfully supported me as we travelled around the region. I often feel they are inconvenienced by my unique situation, yet they are lovingly there by my side helping all the way. Words cannot describe how much I appreciate them.

One of the community initiatives I'm involved in is called Sailability, which provides sailing opportunities for students with special needs and neurodiverse impairments, plus members of the community like me who have a disability. In this context, I need help in order to engage in the experience. But we are also helping others to engage in a sport that is prominent to our country, teaching them skills and having fun at the same time.

This opportunity was first presented to me about 10 years ago by Emily McGowan who was one of my regular support workers at the time. Her father Don McGowan co-founded Sailability with Alan Dick through an international regatta for the Blind Foundation.

To begin the experience, my support worker fits a life jacket on me and secures my daily sling to get me out of the wheelchair. Then, I wheel out to the end of the pier, get winched out of my wheelchair by means of a portable crane secured on the pier, swung around, and dropped down into the sailing dinghy (picture 8).

The Hansa 303 sailing dinghies are equipped with a centreboard keel that is extra weighted for stability. The keel can be raised and lowered depending on the depth of water we launch from. It's a very intimate space with just enough room for the two of us sitting side-by-side on a canvas seat. We have a mainsail and gib which is plenty to enjoy catching the wind.

The first time I went out on the lake, I was ably sailed by a young girl who was blind! Of course, I had no ability to control the boat; she pulled the ropes for the sails and operated the tiller under my direction. I had enough previous sailing experience to be able to do this. There was a lot of trust involved in this experience, but I managed to avoid drowning! It has brought me a lot of pleasure over the years, being so close to the water, out in the elements and active in one of New Zealand's favourite water sports. As Stephen Hawking said, "However difficult life may seem, there is always something you can do and succeed at."[14]

All those who sail have the appropriate safety gear and a handheld radio telephone. I used a normal lifejacket for the first couple of years. Later, I invested in a self-inflating lifejacket which is less bulky and easier to fit on. I decided that it was best to test how this lifejacket works first, and the obvious place to do that was in the rehab pool at Cantabria Lifecare and Village where I used to have regular physiotherapy in the water.

I asked my support workers to fit the lifejacket on me, then hoist me out of my wheelchair and onto the concrete edge of the pool. I instructed Leuila to "just push me in!" She laughed. This would simulate falling out of a boat and into the lake, something I hope to never experience! Debbie remained in the water, while one of the retirement village staff watched from her office right beside the pool. Unlike Leuila, she was somewhat reticent and nervous about this.

In I went, and sank down under the water pretty fast, but I floated up almost immediately as the lifejacket inflated. It tipped me in the upright position, so my head was out of the water. A normal lifejacket leaves me facing head down, so it's quite challenging to rotate upwards in order to breathe properly. I've tested that scenario in the rehab pool as well, managing to lift my head out of the water just enough to catch a breath from time to time!

The self-inflating lifejacket works by dissolving a small tablet in the water, which triggers a gas cartridge, releasing CO_2 into the lifejacket lung. I get the tablet and gas cartridge replaced annually as part of the lifejacket servicing. As you can see, my support workers are called on to help with all kinds of crazy activities!

There are some regular, mundane activities such as going to the doctor or dentist, which I can do on my own, mostly. This is because I can wheel myself there from our home in Lynmore, provided the weather is conducive.

In 2019 I needed a tooth extraction. My regular dentist at

the time felt that it was too tricky for him to tackle. Unlike regular patients, I wheel in beside the dental chair and tilt my chair backwards so the dentist can access my mouth. Occasionally, my dentist will stand on a small stool to reach my mouth.

This particular molar was not easy for him to access, so he referred me to the hospital's dental surgery. I contacted Lakes District Health Board who told me they couldn't help, but suggested I contact one of the local schools which provided some community client work at their dental clinic.

They were not able to help me either, so my dentist referred me to a colleague from Hamilton who ran a weekly clinic in Rotorua at Southern Cross Hospital. He put together a quote for me which I presented to ACC. They had agreed it was fair to fund this treatment on the basis that it wouldn't be an issue if I wasn't in a wheelchair. However, the quote I received created some further discussion.

The total price was $4,878, including the initial consultation, theatre booking, an anaesthetist on standby, surgical removal of the tooth, consumables, medications, and the day recovery room! For goodness' sake, it was only one tooth! If I made my way to the Hamilton clinic, they said they could do the procedure for $2,500.

My ACC case manager was unsurprisingly still keen to explore cheaper options locally. A dentist in Ngongatahā was recommended, so I made an appointment there. During the consultation, the dentist said that he could tackle it on the spot if I wished. I thought, "Why not? Get it dealt with."

It was not an easy extraction, so I was there for just over an hour and the total cost was $195! I simply paid for it and didn't bother getting reimbursed from ACC, who were very happy! I keep my $4,878 tooth in the drawer at home as a memento.

Questions for reflection:

Evaluate the ways in which family and friends have supported you in your journey. Take time to acknowledge them with gratitude and appreciation.

Having read my story, how would you respond differently to families in similar situations to mine?

In the absence of immediate family, who could you adopt to provide support if you are wrestling with an injury that requires their help?

If relevant, rate your experience with ACC. How does it stack up on a scale of 1 to 10? (10 being excellent)

How could you provide support to those living with disability in your own community?

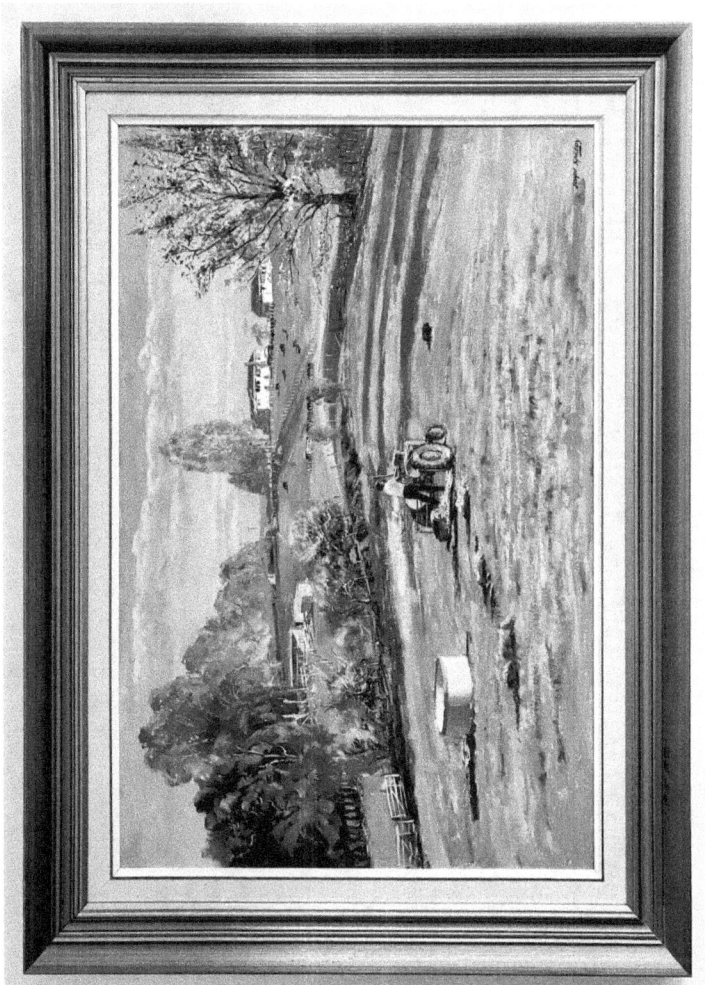

1. A painting of farm life by Tim's uncle John.

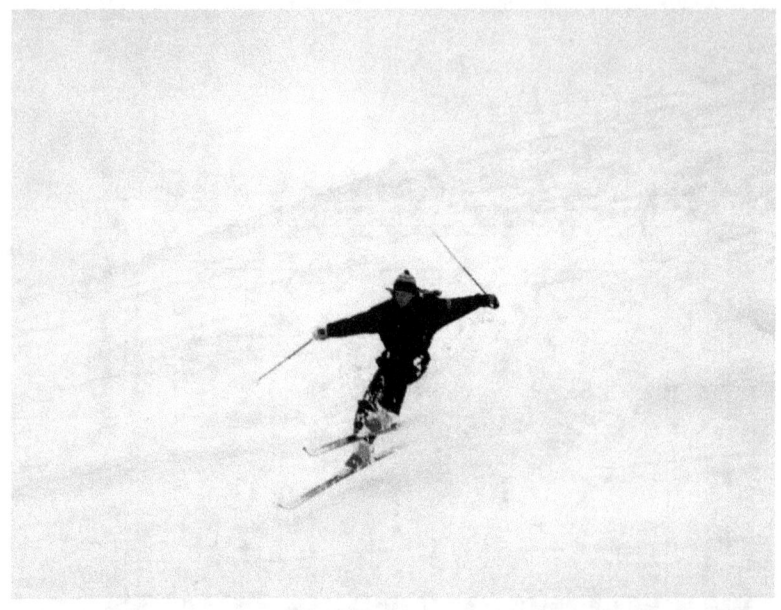

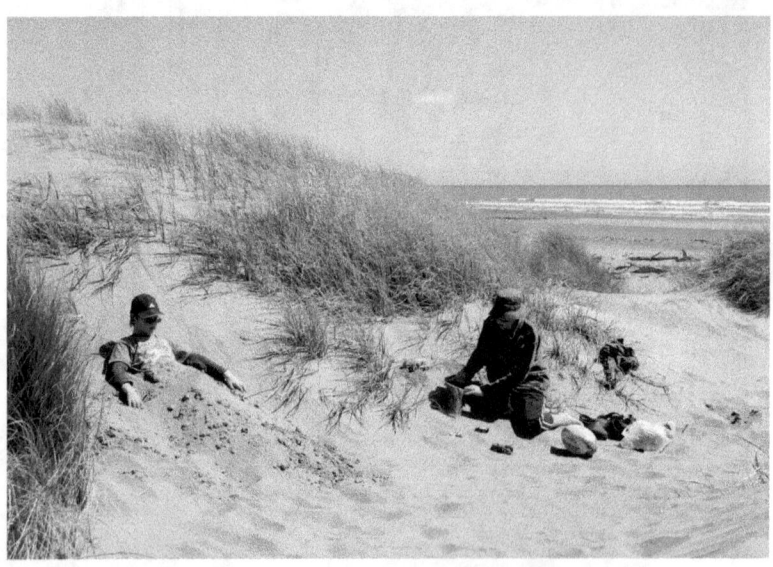

2. Tim skiing in Switzerland, 1991.
3. Hamish and Callum, Waikawa Beach, 2005.

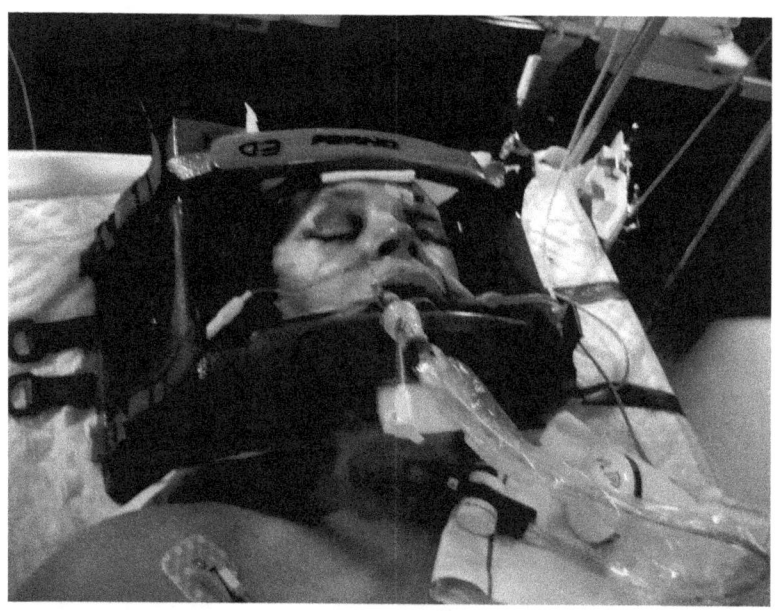

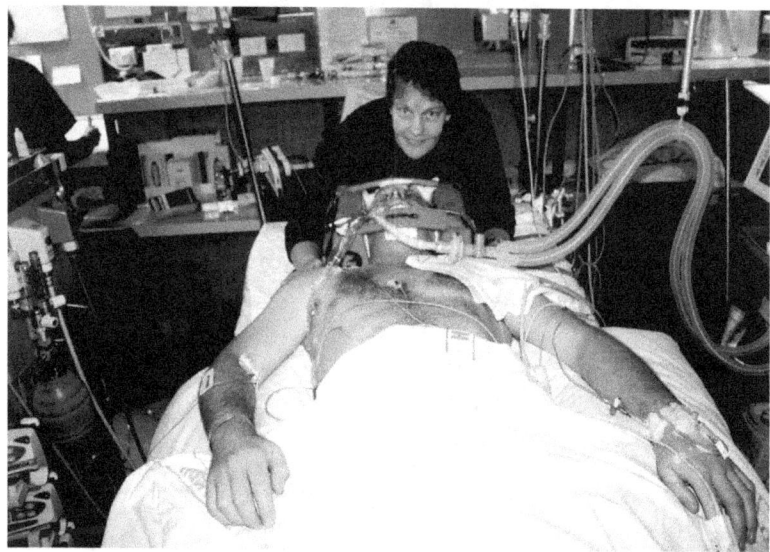

4. In ICU at Rotorua Hospital after the accident.
5. With Jenny.

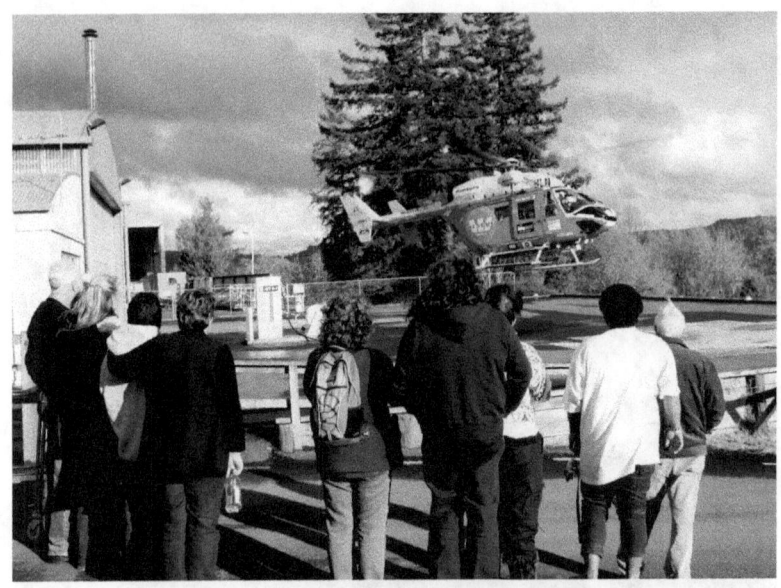

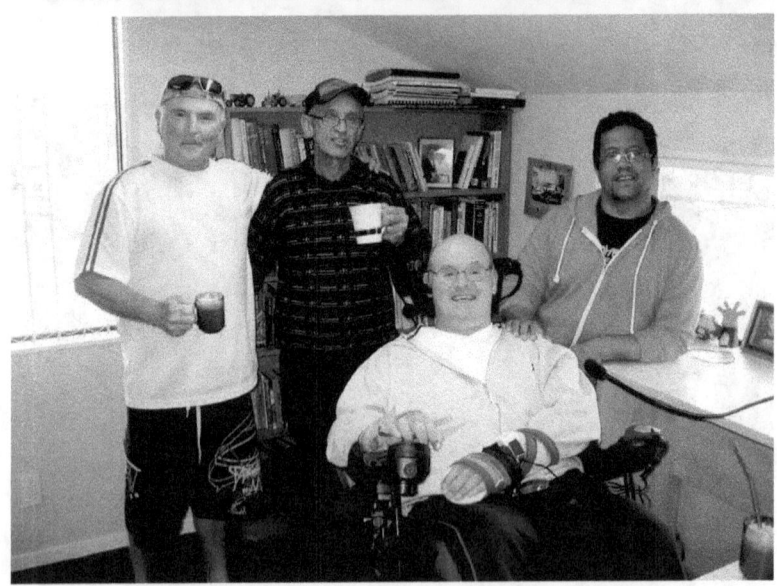

6. Family and friends gather as Tim leaves to Middlemore hospital.
7. First day back in the RBC office, March 2011.

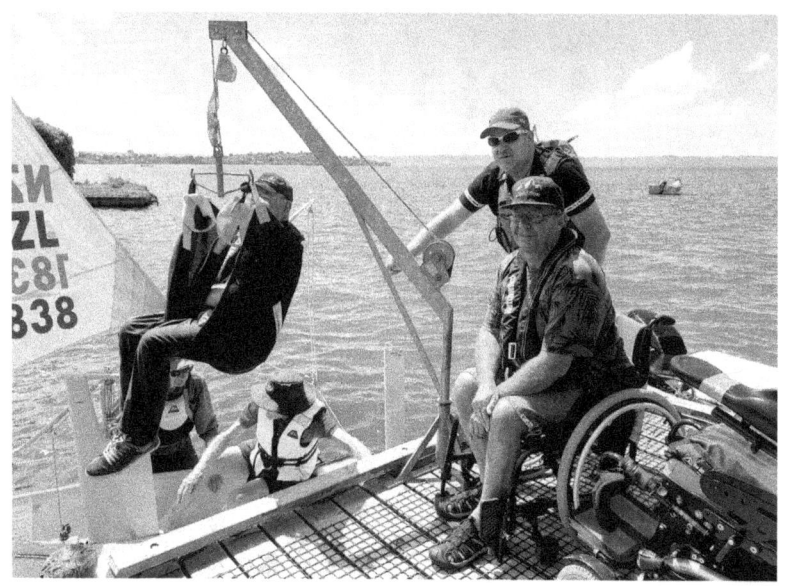

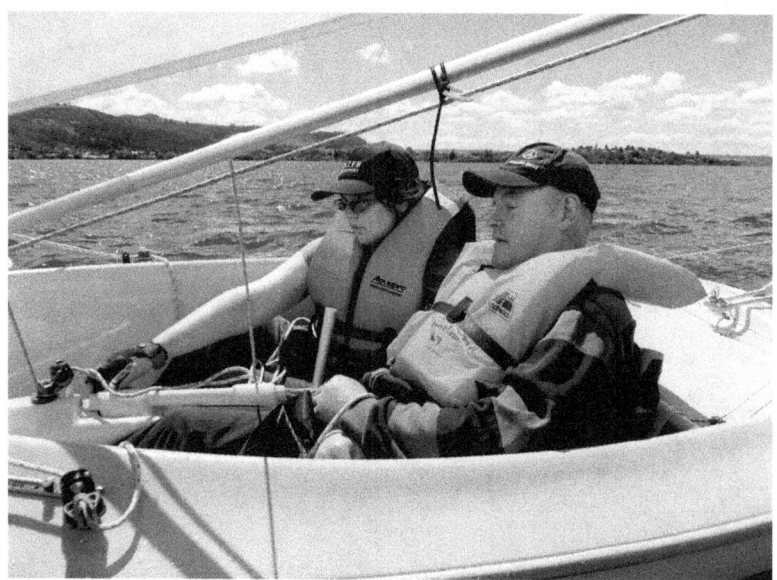

8. Out dinghy sailing with Sailability.

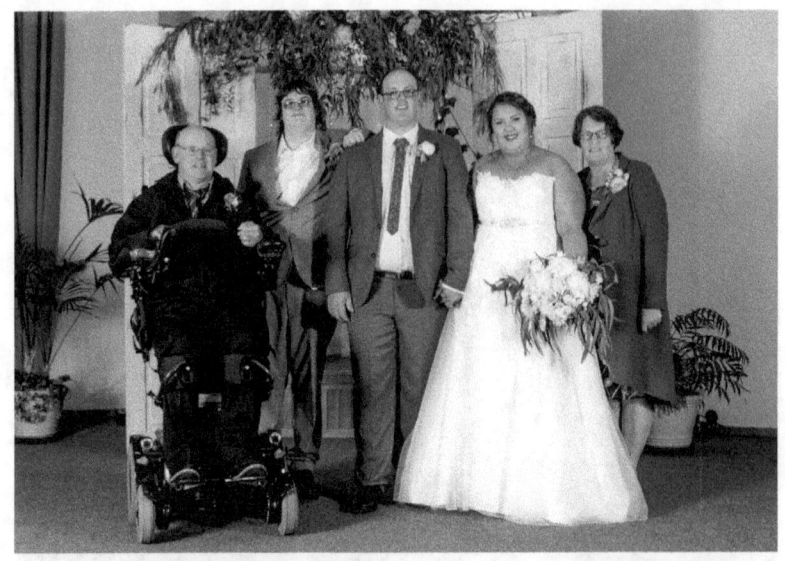

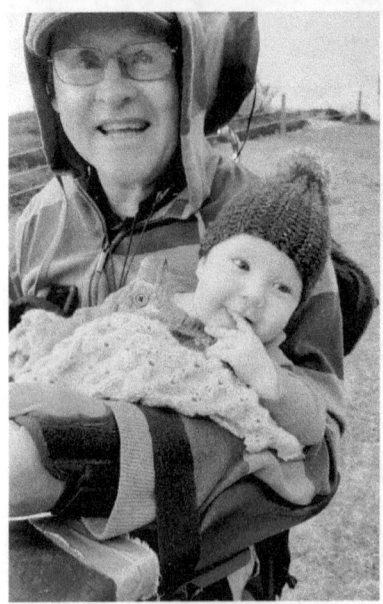
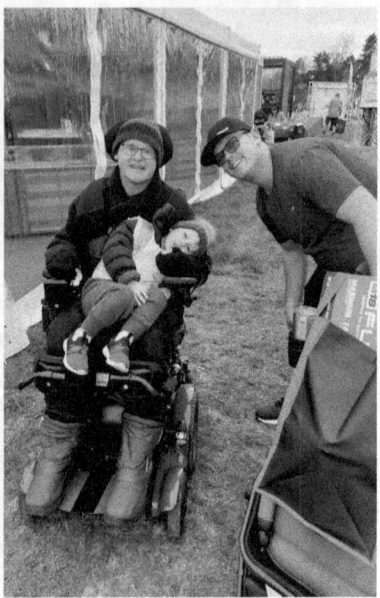

9. The wedding of Hamish and Jess, November 2018.
10. Grandad Tim, with Christopher and Hamish, 2022 and 2024.

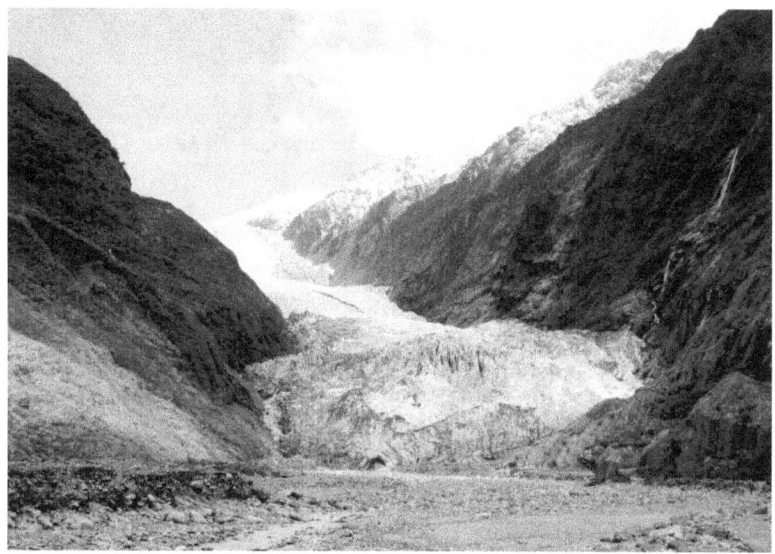

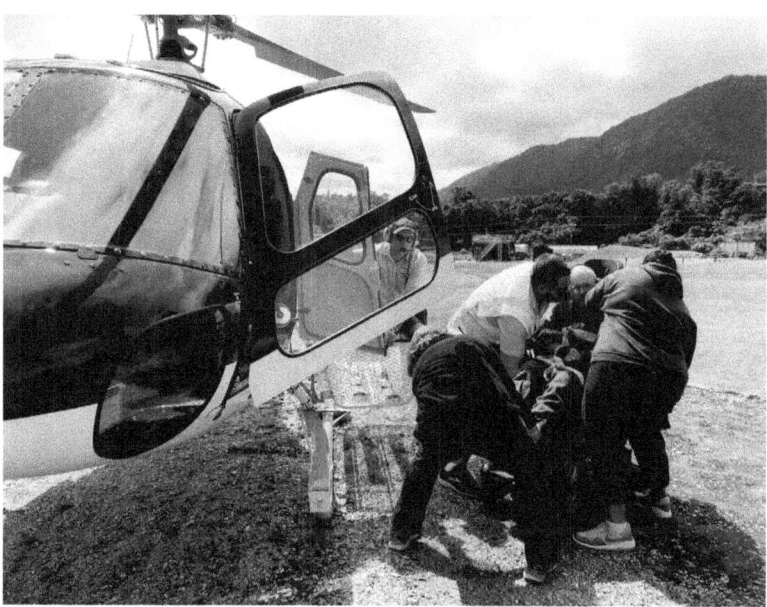

11. *Franz Josef Glacier, February 2020.*
12. *Being lifted into the helicopter.*

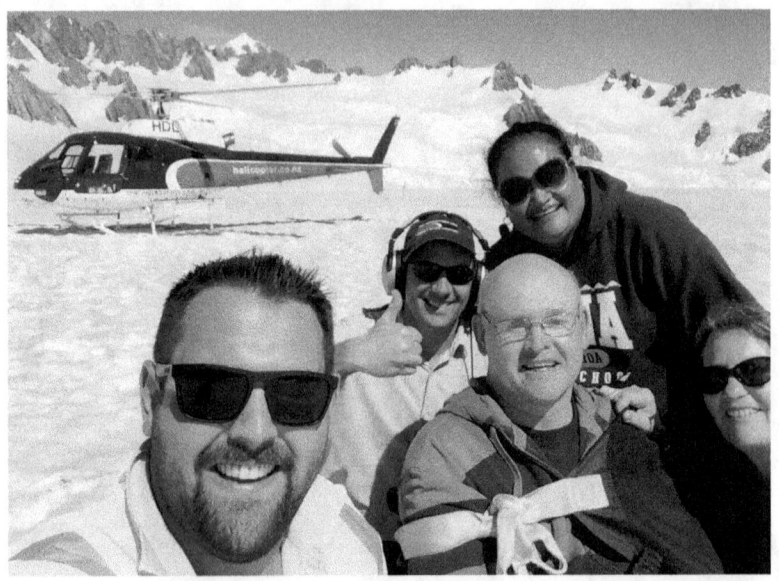

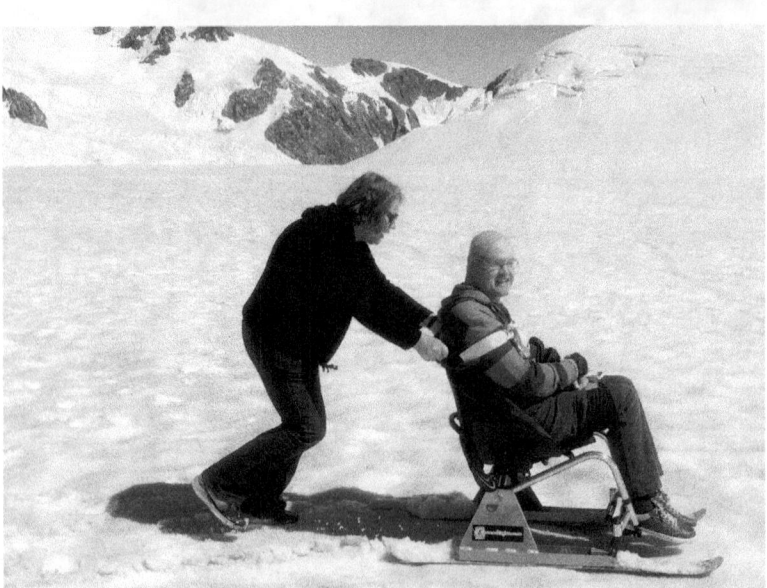

13. Tim at the top of Franz Josef Glacier,
on the snow for the first time since his accident 10 years previously.

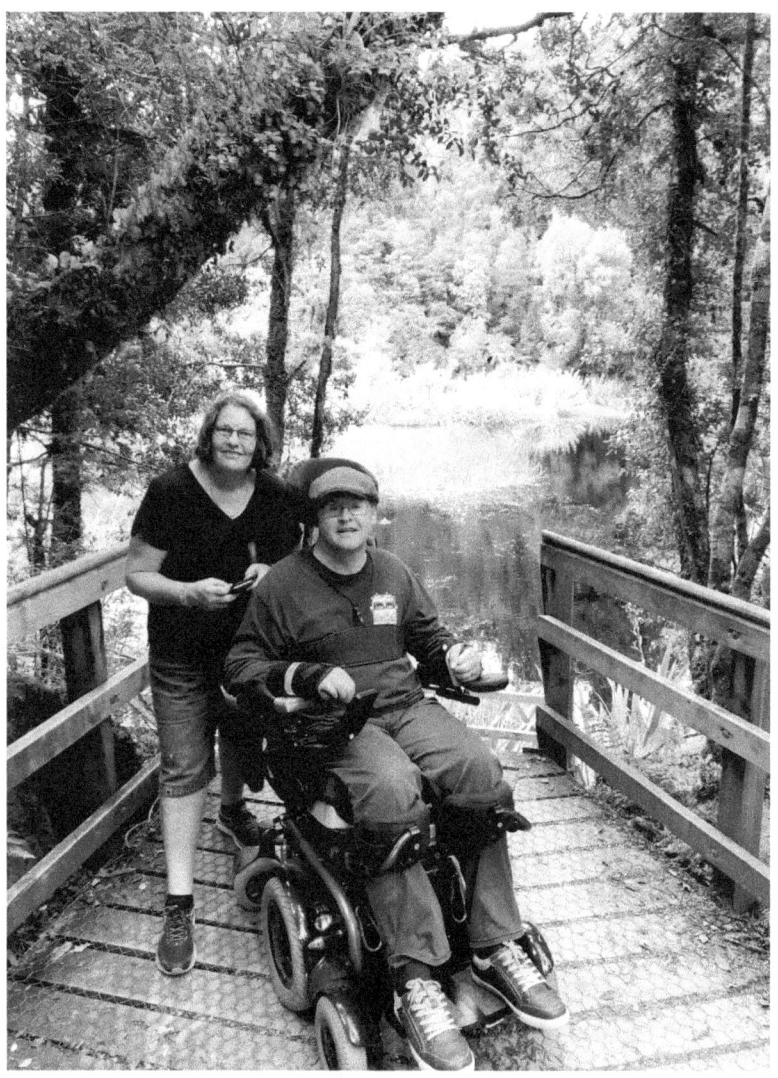

14. *Jenny and Tim at Lake Matheson.*

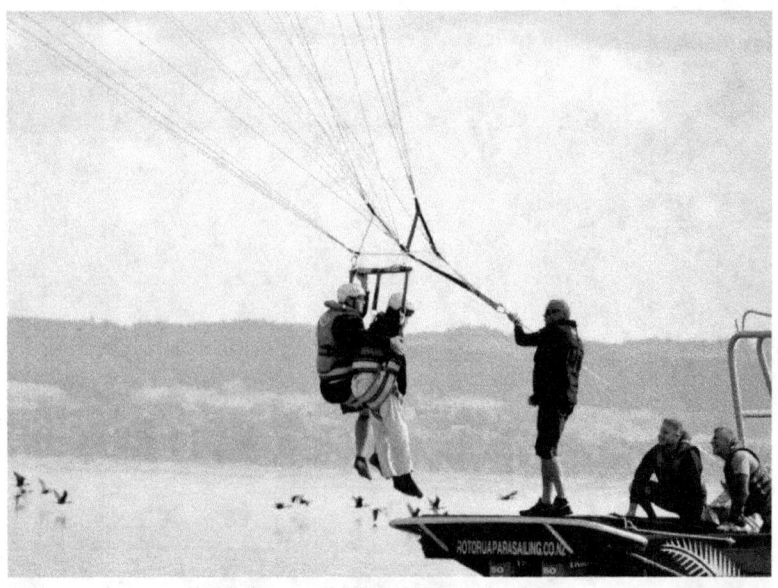
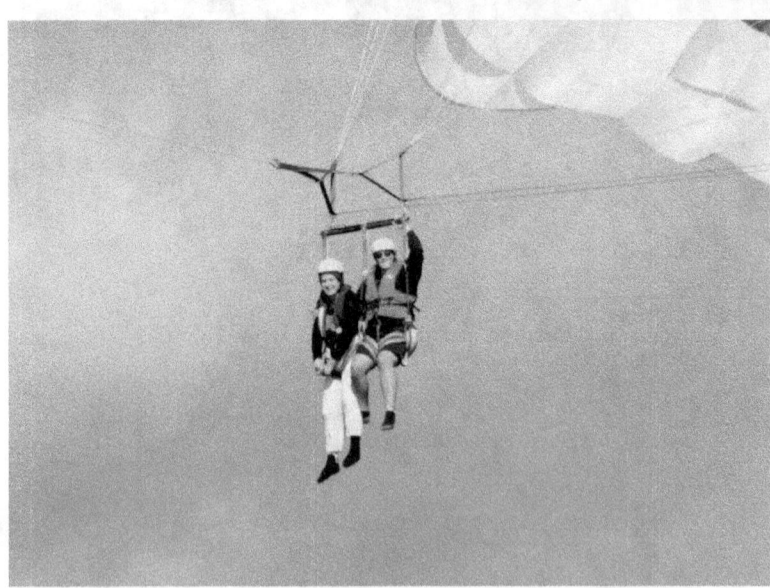
15. Hamish and Tim parasailing over Lake Rotorua, 2016.

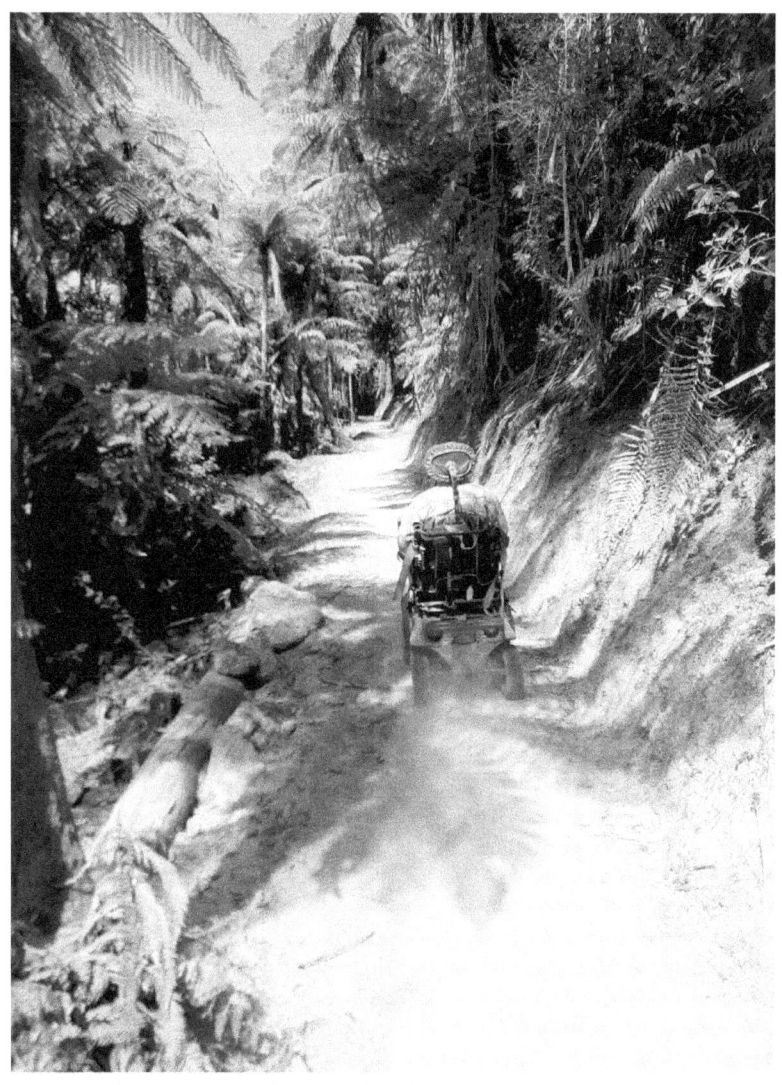

16. *On the forest loop track, January 2022.*

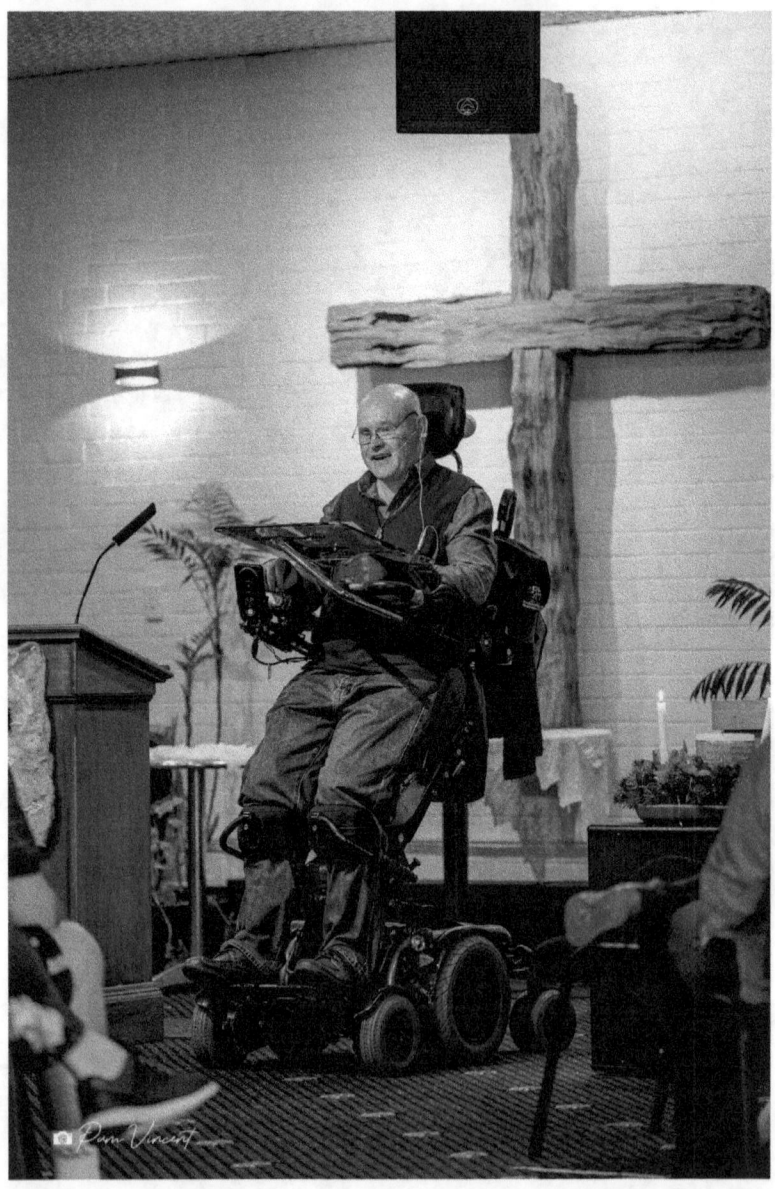

17. Tim preaching at St John's, December 2020.

Chapter 5

Finding My Place in an Unfamiliar World

Accessibility is being able to get into the building. Diversity is getting invited to the table. Inclusion is having a voice at the table. But belonging is having your voice heard at the table!
– Liz Fosslien & Mollie Duffy[1]

Let me tell you about a late friend of mine called Peter Adams. In early 2015, Peter and his wife Joan moved from Whakatane to Rotorua and settled into Ngongotahā village further around the lake from us. Despite Pete, as I used to call him, being older than me, we struck up a friendship. We shared a number of things in common. Pete used to be a lawnmowing contractor and I used to fix lawnmowers. Pete spent several years farming; I grew up on a dairy farm. Pete had a lot of experience operating agricultural machinery; I fixed agricultural machinery for 18 years. There were plenty of down-to-earth practical life stories that we could chat about, and family was always an important topic of conversation. Pete didn't keep good health, basically due to a 'dicky ticker' (fragile heart), so he bought an electric scooter.

There is a disused railway line running from Ngongotahā to the western side of Rotorua. The Rotorua Lakes Council built a sealed walkway alongside it, known as the rail trail. Pete had used his scooter on the rail trail from time to time, and we decided that I could zoom along with him even though he could travel faster than me. I got my support worker to drop me on his side of town, and the aim was to make our way into central Rotorua. We were able to chew the fat on the way while enjoying the countryside together. We did this a few times.

One day I decided to continue through town, out the other side and on to our home 13 kilometres away in the eastern suburb of Lynmore. According to my chair's specifications, I could travel about 20 kilometres, and I figured that my battery should last the distance. Sure enough, it got me home, though I had to coax it along the last few streets by turning the power off and resting it for a few minutes, then powering up and making my way up the hill. Our driveway is quite steep, so I had to call Callum when I reached home, and he gave me a push up.

Sadly, Pete passed away in September 2017. I'm grateful for the brief years we shared together. Joan and I enjoy reminiscing about Pete occasionally when we catch up at Rotorua Baptist Church.

I think it's important to foster relationships across all age groups, cultures, vocational pathways, sporting interests, hobbies, spiritual beliefs and personalities. If everybody is the same colour, we can't make a rainbow, and the world would not be very beautiful if everyone looked like me! Life is the richer for travelling the road with different people and learning from others' experiences. It's important to foster an inclusive atmosphere, thereby reinforcing our diverse culture across multiple contexts.

Some people are difficult to get on with in life, yet they teach us about humility and grace, and they show us that God can use anyone to enrich the world, just as He did in Bible times. The lens by which we see others can be cloudy at times, though.

For example, some people automatically assume that I'm mentally impaired when they see me in an electric wheelchair. In the movie *X-Men Apocalypse*, the main character Xavier is never depicted as being trapped in a wheelchair. His message to the mutants is: "People may think you're a freak or treat you like an outcast, but it doesn't matter what you look like or what people think of you, we will accept you."[2]

People tell me that my personality hasn't changed since the accident, although I'm sure the bang on my head affects my short-term memory from time to time. It's annoying when my recall function is on the blink, though I could probably attribute some of that to old age! Despite the trauma and its impact on my system, I still have my faculties, for which I'm very grateful.

When conversing with me, people realise that I'm still just an ordinary Kiwi bloke who enjoys watching the All Blacks with a cider in hand, celebrating No. 8 wire ingenuity, listening to the sweet sound of a tūī in a kōwhai tree or the burble of a V8 roaring down the road, especially if it's a Maserati! Yes, I admit it; the petrolhead in me remains active in my old age!

Like all New Zealanders, I have interests and passions. However, I am still trying to fit into this world, wrestling with a different set of frustrations in a framework dictated by my spinal injury. As Amanda Lowry says, "You're constantly reminded that you just don't fit. And for lots of people, …it's just too hard."[3]

That said, I can still enjoy our local surroundings in my new circumstances and share the context with other invested parties. For example, I was in the Redwood Forest on my outdoor wheelchair a few years ago, zooming along a fast section of forestry track, when a man pulled up alongside me in his white utility vehicle and wound down the window. "Do you come in here much?" he said. He was one of the Trails Trust staff, responsible for maintenance and development of the mountain bike trails in the park.

The Trust started in 2016 and has grown a lot since then, due to the popularity of the forest for mountain bikers. The Rotorua Lakes Council manages the Trust which operates on tribal (iwi) Māori land. We have 200 kilometres of world-class trails, made more prominent by the Crankworx World Tour, a multi-stop international mountain biking festival which finishes in Rotorua.

I told the man that I was still able to access some of the Grade 2 mountain bike trails (and more recently some of the forest loop track, picture 16). We scheduled a meeting for another day. He also said that they had been improving the tracks with a view to forming an access standard that the local Council can promote for people with disabilities who use adaptive mountain biking equipment or outdoor wheelchairs. That said, I've never seen another crazy person driving an electric wheelchair in the forest, but I hope this will change as time and technology progress!

In February 2023, I was enjoying one of the few sunny days we had in a very wet summer. I sighted the beginning of the Dipper Track and noticed that it had some damage where the rain had scoured it out. Despite that, I was not there to be idle all afternoon. Deciding to take a risk and get on with my adventuring, I entered the track, taking what I considered was the best approach. I quickly found my left-hand wheel sticking up in the air and the remaining drive wheel had lost traction in a rut. I felt sure I was going to tip over and immediately hit the power button in my headrest to the off position. I was careful not to move and prayed with some desperation, "God, would you please bring someone along to help me quickly?"

Somewhere between 10 and 15 minutes later, which seemed like a lifetime, I heard someone walking in the forestry track behind me. I called out and managed to get his attention. He was a tourist, complete with his day pack and map. Soon realising he was from the south side of the English Channel, I drew on my Fourth Form (Year 10) French. "Parlez-vous Anglais, Monsieur?" Sure enough, he knew enough words to help rescue me from my predicament. Off I went, thanking God, and tackling the trail with a greater degree of reticence after a few nervous moments!

This has happened plenty of times, but don't tell my wife that! She has an app called 'Find my iPhone' on her mobile, so she can track wherever I am in the forest. Stink, I can't even escape! I can forgive her from a safety perspective, particularly if I get stuck in some of the more remote places away from regular foot and bike traffic and need to be rescued. Mostly I just want to enjoy the forest on my own, having some solitude in our local paradise. That is why I appreciate having equipment that's been funded to meet my recreational needs.

The company Adapt MTB NZ has all kinds of new equipment suitable for people with a range of disabilities. Most of their equipment has electric capability, coinciding with the many other electric mountain bikes occupying our trails. It's estimated that just over half of New Zealand's 500,000 mountain bikers are riding e-bikes now. My Swiss-made Meyra Optimus 2 RS has more than double the battery capacity of my everyday Levo wheelchair. Therefore, when riding in the forest, I have every confidence it will get me home in time for dinner!

I did come a cropper one Easter, not far from the information centre near the main car park for the Redwoods. There were lots of people coming and going, enjoying walks or rides. I went over a slight mound and ran into a tree, just catching the front left-hand footplate. "Not again," you might say! I swear that tree jumped out in front of me! I wasn't even taking any risks! At the point of impact, my back left-hand trailing wheels rode up over the edge of a punga stump. The combination of the two things happening at the same time was enough to tip the wheelchair over sideways onto the ground.

You'll have to believe me that I wasn't going very fast that time! I was fine, though I felt like a real idiot. I waited for a few minutes then called out, "Is anyone there?" Four lovely ladies appeared, visitors from Auckland for the weekend. "Are you alright, sir?" they asked. They were all occupational therapists! How about that for experts to care for me in those moments? "I'm fine," I said. I gave them directions to pick me back upright, realign my legs and check for any damage to the wheelchair. It was all good. I carried on as if nothing had happened, thanking God for the help I received. I don't believe it was a random thing that four occupational therapists just happened to come to my aid that day; instead, it showed something of God's grace toward me in my hour of need. It's happened too many times to be coincidence!

I encounter people in our community from all different walks of life, each wrestling with different needs and anxieties. Some of them seem quite contented and others are clearly stressed or lonely. Some are open about their lives and others are quite guarded in conversation. If you start digging beneath the surface (many of us stay on a shallow level), you learn that most people are craving a sense of belonging, a place to stand among equals, to simply fit in – their tūrangawaewae. That's where giftedness comes into its own, and our unique identity begins to appear. For some, belonging to a family is enough. Some don't have any family, so a friend or companion becomes that person to include them in life's regular activities, to give them an outlook and a sense of hope. For others, being a member at their local tennis club, library, hobby group, neighbourhood watch, or church group provides a place of belonging. Whether you're an introvert or an extrovert, you can't put a price on knowing that you fit in some way, that you feel valued for your contribution in the community and can simply be yourself without any sense of judgement.

My late friend Andy Valk sought to fit in, despite his previous hard life and the limitations of his blindness. He and his wife Charlene opened their home to strangers at times, extending respite and hospitality to them where possible. This is an honourable practice for any of us to engage in, not forgetting the biblical imperative to,

> *Get into the habit of inviting guests home for dinner or, if they need lodging for the night.* (Romans 12:13b, TLB)

We did this once when we were checking out the neighbours' Christmas lights in their front garden one summer evening. As usual, I was chatting to others around me. One couple were tourists, destined to sleep the night in their car because all the local accommodation was booked out. Considering the lateness of the evening, I invited them home to stay. They felt more comfortable pitching their tent on our back lawn. We offered them a drink, unlocked the back door and said, "Make yourself at home, grab a shower in the morning or whatever you need." Callum was nervous, thinking that they might rob us! But I could see they needed a space to park for the night, somewhere to feel welcome and safe, which of course they were, up our little Lynmore cul-de-sac.

Going back to the story of Andy: He and Charlene moved to Hamilton, but sadly she passed away, leaving Andy alone. I made an effort to see Andy when in Hamilton, often coming away with a sad heart, knowing that he missed Charlene desperately. Each time I left him, he would be sitting in his lounge chair with his seeing-eye dog, Bella, on his lap. He would sit there for hours operating a sound system by voice recognition, much the same as Siri on my iPhone.

I knew he wasn't the easiest character to get along with. Yet he deserved to have a friend, to be treated impartially, and to feel a sense of hope and belonging. I was that person for him, listening to his struggles, laughing at his quirky jokes, and helping him know that he was valued for his contribution to life. Sadly, I wasn't able to attend his funeral when he died. However, I was able to send a couple of stories about our friendship to a family member who shared them with those who gathered to celebrate his life.

I have a book in my office library written by socialist, entrepreneur, speaker and author Joseph R. Myers. He has this to say on the matter:

> *People are trying to find their place in their world, not in individualist ways but in ways that connect. They are searching for a place to belong. They are searching for family. Language may be the key element for developing and nurturing community. As people search for community, they are listening with their eyes, ears and emotions, they are keenly aware of how we tell them they belong or don't belong. People crave connections, not contracts. They want to participate in our rituals, even though they may not yet fully understand their meaning. They see a kaleidoscope of possibilities for belonging.*

But our language struggles to fully express the spectrum of possibilities.[4]

I think Myers' words are insightful and telling; they capture the essence of a two-way relationship, highways going in both directions, channels of learning tinged with grace, opportunities to contribute and receive, to love and be loved, to empathise and recognise synergy in conversation together.

A colleague of mine founded a café in Auckland called Crave. Its philosophy reflects the craving we all have to connect with others, to belong and feel significant. Given the amount of patronage we witnessed when we visited once, it's apparent that locals in the community feel very much at home, conversing freely in that environment.

We all have something to give in life, be it in word or deed. I believe that God has kept me alive to encourage my fellow humans, to give hope and to inspire others whenever and wherever the opportunity presents itself. Every conversation and relationship I have is fulfilling for me, no matter the context or time invested. Whether I am supporting people pastorally, interacting with a neighbour or supervising colleagues over a cup of coffee, we meet as gifted individuals, sharing life in the moment, enriched through a sense of belonging for the time shared.

This Māori whakataukī (proverb) says it well:

Nāku te rourou, nāu te rourou, ka ora ai te iwi. With your food basket and my food basket, the people will thrive. This whakataukī talks to community, to collaboration and resourcefulness, to a strengths-based approach in life. It acknowledges that everybody has something to offer, a piece of the puzzle, and by working together we can all flourish.[5]

A world devoid of meaningful two-way relationships is a world devoid of learning, of shared experience, of the ability to understand love in the context of joy or suffering. Amanda Lowry lives in the nearby city of Tauranga and shares a similar journey to mine, having sustained a spinal injury in a surfing accident. To her credit, she is using that journey to help others feel more included in her local context and beyond. She advocates for others with mobility issues and consults at the Tauranga City Council. She also swims and serves on the International Paralympic Committee. She says: "Lived experience locates our understandings of the world."[6]

How many people without hope are trying to exit this world through tragic and avoidable suicidal pathways because they can't interpret life as they know it through the lens of healthy relationships, hope, and experiences where diversity is celebrated and free of prejudice? According to Health New Zealand, in the 2023/24 financial year, there were 617 suspected self-inflicted deaths in Aotearoa New Zealand.[7] How many of these deaths could be avoided if people felt they belonged and stood as one among equals?

I'm involved with a local community group whose members have a range of different life experiences and disabilities. One chap who comes to our meetings has an irritating, high-pitched whining voice, a tendency to go off topic, often complains instead of focusing on solutions, and talks so much that people start rolling their eyes. He even carries a wooden spoon around in his bag and calls himself a 'stirrer'! However, he finds a sense of belonging in our group and is a reminder of the grace we must extend to each other, despite a level of frustration and the interruption to our own agenda. If he didn't have a voice, he wouldn't have much hope in addressing the issues that are important to the community in which he lives in and for whom he advocates.

An inclusive society doesn't just affect the way we communicate and treat each other; it also extends to accessibility. In March 2016, I enrolled in a three-day mentoring/coaching course at a venue in Auckland. One week before the course was due to start, the facilitator contacted me to say that they had booked an upstairs room in a church which had no lift. Thankfully, he realised that I couldn't attend, apologised and assured me that a suitable venue would be available for the next course. Imagine if I had arrived, only to discover I was excluded, had to turn around and go home.

I had a similar experience another time when I was officiating at a friend's wedding ceremony in November 2022. While the hosts were friendly, the owner of the venue was less than accommodating. Reception venues were limited at that time and the couple kindly asked if I was able to access the wedding breakfast venue, knowing that the local hotel had quite dated facilities, notably the reception room which had stairs at the entry off the footpath.

I consulted with venue staff about access several months before the event. I could use my two-metre portable ramps to navigate steps up to the porch, but another step to the right made further access difficult. They were quite nice but made it clear that the owner of the building was not interested in permanently improving access to their facility, "as it may hinder others' movements when attending wedding functions." I would have thought that an accessible entrance helped mitigate the risk of intoxicated guests falling and injuring themselves or others in the process! Their reasoning was clearly flawed!

After some discussion, they did at least build a temporary

ramp for the top step, and I made it inside. On the day of the wedding, just after I gained access to the reception venue, another chap in a manual wheelchair followed behind us. Fortunately for him, he was able to use my ramps to gain access, along with an elderly person using a walker. Imagine how challenging it would have been for them if I wasn't there with my equipment.

When it came time to leave, we offered to leave my ramps set up for the other chap to use when he left. We indicated that we could pick them up from him after the event. He seemed like a trustworthy person. He was grateful but insisted that we take our ramps with us and that it wasn't our responsibility to compensate for the poor access to the venue. He said that he would make a scene with the hotel staff when leaving, hoping it would challenge their views on accessibility! Did I expect that to make a difference? Probably not.

More recently, I was asked to consult with a group, visiting some of the hotels in Rotorua. The purpose of our tour was to see how accessible their accommodation suites and function rooms were. Our team leader was hosting the biannual Oceania Seating Symposium, and many of the 300 delegates from around the globe required accessible rooms due to their mobility needs.

We discovered that many of the rooms were unsuitable, with insufficient space to park equipment like wheelchairs and commodes, little room around the bed, narrow entranceways, tight corners and uneven entrances into bathrooms. Not one of the beds had sufficient clearance underneath to accommodate the legs of a hoist for lifting people from bed to wheelchair and back again.

Most of the hotel staff were warm and friendly, happy to show us around and answer our questions. To our amazement, we learnt that some of the rooms had been recently refurbished, yet they were still not suitable. Staff were aware of the need for accessible rooms, but clearly had not consulted people with lived experience like me. Some noted they had never been asked about the things we raised with them. They responded to us with silence, clearly not interested in making the necessary changes for rooms to be truly accessible and inclusive. Universal design means that it should suit everybody, but our experience showed that neither staff nor contractors were au fait with the appropriate standards. However, I will keep on chipping away, seeking to educate and coax people to think more inclusively – it's a hard gig!

ACC have what they call 'family enhancement', which stems from policies that deal with treatment of family members and housing modifications.[8] The term embraces a financial commitment to meet each client's complex needs, including accessibility to places of residence, vocation and, in some cases, social or recreational contexts. In my case, they installed a lift in our house which gave me the ability to access all three levels of our home.

City councils and workplaces are slowly catching on, building public facilities with accessible bathrooms, ramps, and seating areas big enough to accommodate users plus their friends or family members. In my capacity as a member of the Rotorua Access Group for CCS Disability Action, together with fellow wheelchair users, I've consulted with Rotorua Lakes Council (RLC) on several projects over the years.

The most recent one is to improve the facilities at nearby Lake Tarawera. Adjacent to the café/restaurant is a newly developed car park and lakeside picnic area which has been designed to accommodate people with mobility needs. The picnic tables have added room for wheelchairs to pull up alongside other users, and the toilets are also designed for easy access.

Another project I previously collaborated on is the wider footpath down Tītokorangi Drive (formerly Long Mile Drive) which accesses nearby forest walking tracks and mountain bike trails. We lobbied for two years to also include a safety refuge in the middle of Tarawera Road. More recently it has been upgraded to a full crossing, and the Council has included another safety refuge higher up the road near our street. This makes it safer for me to cross when accessing the Redwoods in my outdoor wheelchair.

I've been party to discussions for the newly developed Queen Elizabeth Health facility which opened in February 2023, and for the upgraded Rotorua Aquatic Centre which opened in June 2024. I'm collaborating with the staff at QE Health to ensure they acquire the necessary equipment for people with a range of mobility issues to be able to use their facilities. Even in my role as a volunteer chaplain at Rotorua Hospital, I've been able to negotiate with grounds staff to have outside seating areas with extra room for people with wheelchairs and walkers.

Our Access Group brief extends to road crossings and bus routes as well. For example, I'm not able to reach out my arm and press the button to stop traffic at a pedestrian crossing. So, New Zealand Transport Agency Waka Kotahi engineers and Council reps invited me to consult with them on the best possible way to safely cross busy traffic. As a result, they have installed a proximity sensor, which means I can draw close to the roadside pole and stop traffic to safely cross the road without having to push the button.

All my efforts at a community level are with others in mind, such as elderly people with scooters, parents with children in pushchairs, and people with impaired hearing or eyesight. I've been privileged, along with other community members with vested interests, to help develop a new accessibility policy; Stage I was signed off by Council in April 2025.

It sometimes takes years of lobbying to improve accessibility in our community infrastructure, but I'm thrilled to see results which promote inclusivity for everyone. Council IT staff have contacted me to help improve their systems and online survey platforms so that people using assistive technology can easily have input on what's happening at a local level. When many surveys are done online, it's useful to know that the Council here is taking an inclusive approach for our demographic.

We will always find things to complain about in terms of Council debt and decision-making that impacts us directly, but I wish to give them some credit where it's due! The members I work with are passionate about their roles, and I enjoy collaborating with them for the sake of our community, and the many visitors we have, nationals and internationals. In an article for the *Rotorua Daily Post*, journalist Maryanna Garcia wrote, "Councils have a minimum requirement, and developers are required to meet basic standards but some of those requirements are actually inadequate."[9]

Sometimes, inaccessibility in public places can lead to embarrassing moments. Once, when Callum and I were out together on a Thursday afternoon, we stopped to have our usual cup of coffee plus a lemon, lime and bitters at the Columbus coffee shop in Rotorua's central mall. I know the owner – a lovely Chinese man called Edison.

It was just on closing time, and they were cleaning up, but Edison invited us in from the street entrance. He moved a table and sign in front of the door, but there was a lip to negotiate.

As I lurched over the top of the lip, the bump set my muscles into spasm and I drove forward at speed, running into the table, knocking the sign onto the ground and sending Edison and his staff scattering in all directions! Fortunately, no one else was in the café at the time, so humiliation was kept to a minimum! Callum and I proceeded to sit down at a table outside and laughed while waiting for our drinks. 'The Old Man' can be hugely embarrassing at times, as Callum reminds me on occasion!

The challenge is for those who manage the mall to ensure better, level entrances to shops, and access across car parks. Along with a fellow wheelchair user, I have met with those who oversee these specific public areas. At one such meeting in late 2023, I learnt that some of the issues we raised had been discussed as far back as 2015 and had still not been addressed! Alas, the wheels turn slowly, but at least we are trying.

Occasionally I attend public events like rugby games or concerts, and I'm pleasantly surprised at the good level of access available. My friend Rob Powley took me to a Bob Dylan concert at Claudelands Event Centre in Hamilton. We had the best seats in the house! I've met with the staff at our local rugby stadium, and they are seeking to improve the very outdated facilities there. It's a work in progress, but I'm glad to play a part on behalf of our community and its members.

In my capacity as a preacher, I am privileged to speak and minister to all kinds of people in different contexts. Over the years I have spoken at national and regional camps for the Elevate Christian Disability Trust. They do a fantastic job – raising awareness, educating church groups, and promoting wellbeing and inclusiveness for people with disabilities. Former director Di Willis is the most powerful and effective advocate

I've ever met. Her heart and passion towards those who are less fortunate is second to none. The welcome message on the Elevate website states:

> *Since 1975 we have been empowering people with disabilities to live to their full potential – physically, mentally, socially and spiritually. We create places of belonging, hope and encouragement through branches around New Zealand.*[10]

I was speaking at an Elevate camp in West Auckland in April 2017, promoting family, what it means to belong together, and how that is encouraged within biblical and Christian frameworks. At the end of my first session, I offered prayer to those in attendance. A young Chinese man with cerebral palsy who had a great sense of humour and a demeanour of contentment, came forward. I found him very difficult to understand but he asked, "Could I help you pray for people?" I said, "Sure," thinking to myself that people would really struggle to comprehend him. As they came forward, he laid his hands on them, and I prayed. Each of us did what the other one couldn't. It was one of the most powerful things I have ever experienced.

> *Each of you should use whatever gift you have received to serve others, as faithful stewards of God's grace in its various forms.* (1 Peter 4:10)

When preaching, I'm able to educate people from the perspective of lived experience. The use of language and how we define people with disabilities can be disempowering if articulated flippantly. For example, when I booked a motel for one summer holiday, the woman on the phone described her accessible unit as the 'disabled room'. This is no different from talking about a 'disabled car park', or 'disabled toilets'. It's very demeaning. Despite my efforts to educate her, she wouldn't entertain thinking or conversing in a different manner. After she cut me down abruptly, I concluded that it was too hard for her to think about changing the way she spoke.

Regional councils tend to use the term 'mobility car parks', along with the well-known symbol of someone in a wheelchair. That's a step in the right direction. Why shouldn't we use softer language to describe users while keeping their true identity associated with character, values, heritage and culture, as I've mentioned before?

If we use our language in a more empowering way, we can acknowledge the ways people with unique needs and disabilities contribute to the community, despite appearances or demeanour. Everyone should be given equal opportunity to serve and be valued for their contribution, even if it seems minimal. In my experience, people with few social skills often relish the opportunity to help in some way. It puts a smile on their face.

According to the 2013 New Zealand Disability Survey, an estimated 1.1 million New Zealanders (24 percent) had some form of disability.[11] That's an awful lot of fellow Kiwis we should be making life easier for!

I believe that all of us are created in the image of God, though some of us take a while to discover the unique talent or gift that helps us make sense of the world in which we live. The Church is one of many groups and institutions within our communities that needs to make an effort to include people with unique needs.

Theologian Myk Habets has written:

People with disabilities gift the church with a different way of being human together. In this vision, limitations, dependence and vulnerability are normal parts of being human, therefore power and self-determination equal cultural ideals that limit our witness to the gospel.[12]

When using the metaphor of the body, the apostle Paul commended his readers to give extra honour and care to the vulnerable and marginalised parts, seeking to bring harmony among members of the Church in the Greco-Roman world (1 Corinthians 12:23-25). After all, don't our bodies function better when all the parts work together in a healthy fashion? Not seeking honour for myself, I do feel an added responsibility to look out for those who are marginalised in our culture. Together, we make for a richer and more balanced Kiwi society, including the Church.

Charles Hewlett, National Leader of the Baptist Churches of New Zealand, authored a book with his wife Joanne called *Hurting Hope: What parents feel when their children suffer*. The book tells their story of living with two children who have profound disabilities. Charles reflects on the wonderful ways in which their local church has treated them as a family, yet he is honest about the fact that churches can do better about inclusion and accessibility. Murray Sheard from the Christian Blind Mission (CBM) reflected in a podcast with Charles that we just don't 'see' people with disabilities in the Church. He asks what churches can do better to include members with disabilities. During that podcast, Charles said:

Maybe it's time to reconsider who participates in the mission of God; just broaden the definition of participation... How might our mission agencies be different if we grasped this? Just be brave, treat them with respect, be genuine and honest. For people who see them as healing objects – they will fade away. Those who see them as genuine will be there for the long haul... Work hard at seeing them beyond the dribble, beyond the wheelchair... Take a risk, be a friend to them. Inform the church about them, involve them, be sacrificial.[13]

In my first year as senior pastor at Rotorua Baptist Church, while I was preaching one Sunday morning, a young boy got up out of his seat and wandered forward onto the stage. He banged the drum kit briefly and roamed around in front of us until his mum came and directed him back to their seat. I eyeballed his mum and reassured her not to worry, then informed the congregation that this young boy had some unique needs that we should accommodate. His mum smiled at me and people relaxed. I know from experience that the young boy had autism and is what's known as 'a runner'.

It's far better to celebrate and embrace some disruption and noise from children in church, rather than have people turn their heads and display grumpy body language at the parents or caregivers. After all, are we not a family, journeying and learning together as young and old, introvert and extrovert, Kiwi and immigrant, etc? I'm pleased to say that our current pastoral leaders at Rotorua Baptist Church are on board with this, making it known to the congregation on a regular basis. It's about fostering an inclusive culture which speaks volumes to those who may be exposed to the life of the church. This principle extends to whatever community group or organisation we may be part of. As Di Willis said, "A church that doesn't have disabled people in it, is a disabled church... I sometimes say that if the church was really doing its job, we wouldn't need this ministry [Elevate] at all."[14]

All communities would thrive better and be more fruitful if we could accommodate each other's uniqueness and work together for the better of our fellow humans. One of the finalists in the 2015 Pride of New Zealand awards, Jim Edwards, helps rehabilitate accident victims with his 40-seater waka. Paddling, steering, haka, chants, greeting strangers, photography, doing maintenance, and being able to kōrero all help the rehabilitation process. He also teaches adults with disabilities how to use their hands as well as their minds, with other skills including carving, vehicle restoration and gardening. In a *New Zealand Herald* article, he likened life to a waka which we're all in together, holding our paddles, or hoe, on the great river: "When you all hoe, you hoe together. If you all work together, you achieve your goals."[15]

I applaud Jim's philosophy, having had first-hand experience of riding in a waka at nearby Lake Ōkāreka in 2006, when I came to Rotorua as a parent help for our son's school camp. One of the organised experiences for the students was to paddle a waka together. This teaches the value of working together as a group to achieve their goals. As part of canoe skills (waka ama), they learn about culture, leadership, teamwork, respect, and most importantly the value of inclusion.

We were all seated side-by-side in the waka. Off we went. As we moved through the settled waters of the lake, the leader or caller (kaihautū) at the front instructed us to paddle (hoe) in unison. We called out 'kaihoe hī', which means 'be ready' each time we scooped our paddles in the water. I noticed the Māori girl sitting next to me expressing these words and actions with great passion. That sense of synergy with the experience was inspiring.

As we made our way across the lake, turned corners and chanted battle cries, our leader included the word 'togetherness' and the phrase 'no passengers' in his instructions to us. The Māori proverb (whakataukī) "He waka eke noa" reflects the full intent of his words; it means "We're all in this together."[16]

I have these words on the number plate of our van. They have become a key factor in my philosophy of pastoral ministry and leadership, and were the seed of my calling to the senior pastor role at Rotorua Baptist Church back in 2008. They speak to the apostle Paul's calling to reach the Gentile people who were once separated from the Jews and estranged from the gospel (Ephesians 2:11-22). The essence of Jesus Christ's ministry was to bring peace and reconciliation for mankind, to bridge the gap between cultures, to cut through man-made divisions and foster the same kind of togetherness that our caller was instilling in us on the boat. In my opinion, this is one of the reasons why we should uphold the tenants of Te Tiriti o Waitangi, because New Zealand's founding treaty agreement was forged to bring fairness, respect and unity among cultures.

When everyone is working together toward the same horizon, anything is possible – for individuals, communities and countries alike. If such were the case, there'd be no hint of war, hatred or bitterness, but rather, the ever-pervasive values of love, unity and oneness. Perhaps this is what is behind another well-known Māori proverb: "He aha te mea nui o te ao? He tangata he tangata he tangata." ("What is the most important thing in the world? It is people. It is people. It is people.")[17]

As mentioned in Chapter 1, my calling into pastoral ministry was established out of a deep and sincere love for people, and a desire to journey with them, either in brief encounters, for a season or for an extended period of time. For example, in my capacity as a pastor, I've taken a significant number of funerals over the years and supported many families through times of illness and bereavement.

Here is a humorous anecdote to conclude this chapter. On one occasion, I was visiting one of my parishioners in Rotorua, a lovely lady called Hazel Williamson. She was on her deathbed, so I popped around to visit her at home. Hazel's husband Alex opened the front door and invited me in. The door was just wide enough for my electric wheelchair, although I had to navigate an aluminium lip at the base, approximately 40 millimetres high. Many people's front doors are like this, which is why I often go in through the garage if they have level entry into their homes. It's tricky getting over lips because I have to operate the joystick with just enough force to get both wheels acting in unison.

As I went over the lip with some momentum, the wheelchair skewed slightly left and squashed Alex's finger up against the wall behind the door. Poor Alex limped back to the lounge dripping blood on the carpet. His daughter attended to him, and you can imagine how I felt as I made my way to Hazel's bedroom to pray and sing with her. We laughed about it after the event! Some years later when taking Alex's funeral, I was chatting to his wife's daughter from a previous marriage. She told me that the doorknob still had a dent in it!

Questions for reflection:

What does it mean for you to feel included?

How are you making a difference for others, perhaps by giving them a job to do in your business, organisation, club or church?

In what ways could you influence your local politicians or council to ensure the needs of people with disabilities are better met?

Is there a balanced representation of people in your church leadership team? If not, how might you change this?

How can your church better accommodate the demographic of your community?

Chapter 6
Where is God When Bad Things Happen?

The deepest pain asks the best questions.
– William P. Young, author of *The Shack*[1]

In this chapter, I will attempt to address the issue of suffering and injustice, looking more deeply into the things we have no easy answers for and the reality that a loving God seems so distant at times. Yet, in the darkest places, where grief and uncertainty lie, I believe hope and fortitude are within reach for all of us, helping us to survive the rigours of life in the 21st century.

Having a spinal injury creates an added dimension of vulnerability for me. For example, it's not easy being ill and needing somebody to blow my nose, clear congestion, catch my vomit, change my position in bed when my legs are aching with nerve pain, or when they spasm vigorously, waking Jenny and me at 2am. Temperature regulation is difficult to manage as well. I'm not even sure whether I feel hot or cold at times! This makes it challenging to know how many layers of clothing to put on, or what bedding to use. It takes time and effort to rectify these things with my family or support workers; things that most of us take for granted.

If I am sick or have a pressure sore that is not healing quickly enough, then I have no choice other than to rest in bed. As I am an active person who likes to get on with life, you can imagine the mental challenge it is for me being laid up in bed for even a couple of days. I can empathise to some degree with a couple of gentlemen I know here in the Bay of Plenty, both of whom have spinal injuries and have been stuck in bed for at least three and a half years, sometimes dealing with significant pressure sores. One of them is retired and faces the prospect of seeing out most of his remaining years stuck in bed.

Watching Mr Bean on YouTube, Netflix movies, or car shows on TV is a great distraction when I am unwell. These activities go some way in helping to mask my internal pain and grief as well. For others, the grief of losing someone can be softened by applying the same strategy. As grief and bereavement expert, Dr Camille Wortman, wrote,

> It is certainly clear from the research evidence, as well as from my own personal life, that distraction can be an important element in the mourning process. Yet almost nobody talks about it![2]

Sometimes TV shows are a mixed blessing. The mechanic in me enjoys watching programmes on classic car restoration. It's amazing how vehicles destined for the scrap yard can be saved. Yet frustration is never far from my thoughts, if I'm honest. I often think of times before my accident when I could hook the trailer onto the back of my car and help someone move house. Or, as a pastor, take someone down to the petrol station to fill up their tank with fuel, load up someone's grocery trolley, or hop in the car late in the evening to spend time with someone in a relationship crisis. These things are no longer possible for me and that generates feelings of grief that well up inside me regularly. It feels like a big part of my being has gone through a death experience.

Furthermore, responding to my family's practical needs is challenging, even now, more than a decade after my bike accident. Several months after Hamish moved into his own home across town, a young man stole a car in the middle of the night, sped down Fairy Springs Road, lost control of his vehicle and ran off the road into Hamish's property.

Hamish woke up, thought it was an earthquake and went back to sleep! When he woke up again some minutes later, he heard the noise of rushing water. He got up and discovered the offender's car sitting in a mangled state across his driveway. It had ploughed into a power pole, through the boundary fence two doors down, then bounced over the neighbours' front concrete porch, scraped the soffit above that, flown over the adjoining boundary fence and smacked right into the kitchen wall at the front corner of Hamish's house before settling on the driveway.

The impact shunted the fridge across the dining room, through the door and into the lounge. Water was spouting from dislodged plumbing and exposed electrical wires presented sufficient risk for Hamish to exit the house and contact emergency services. The offender had left their vehicle and run off up the street. Police soon located them – injured and guilty!

Hamish tried calling me several times until I eventually woke up. I couldn't jump out of bed and answer the phone like most people; instead, I called out to my support worker who was asleep in the room next door. I desperately wanted to head downstairs to the garage and go to my son's aid as soon as possible. It's my job to rescue my son, but that wasn't going to happen, and it made me angry.

He was able to reach Jess, his girlfriend at that time, who was at home with her mum not far away. After a brief while she came to see him for moral support. It does my head in not being able to immediately respond and offer practical help whenever an urgent need presents itself, especially for my family. The injustice of my spinal injury is too much to bear some days. I can relate to this description from *TIME* magazine: "What makes spinal cord injuries as devastating as they are is that everything about them plays out in absolutes: they are instantaneous, utterly disabling and horribly permanent."[3]

I was at least able to call Hamish back and assure him that I would make it across town to see him as soon as my support worker got me up. It gave me a little hope to be able to process the event with him and welcome him back home to stay with us until his property was assessed and repaired. He had only been in his own house about four months. The insurance payout enabled him to upgrade the kitchen and improve the layout of the dining room, so that was a blessing in disguise.

Hamish is still working through renovations in his home and property, jointly owned with Jess, who is now his wife. I desperately wish I could pick up a hammer and join him to speed up the process. Any opportunity to at least discuss what he's working on is an absolute pleasure for me, not to mention organising parts and helping him with maintenance on his GMC truck!

As a pastor, I've been in touch with plenty of people who are coping with their own sufferings in life. In 2017 I was preaching out of town at another Baptist church when a couple asked me to pray with them after the service. The husband had some blood vessels in his head cauterised as a form of treatment for atrial fibrillation. As a result of this procedure, he had suffered a severe stroke and could not walk or talk properly anymore.

The doctor told him it was bad luck, given that only one percent of patients who have this procedure is adversely affected. Not very encouraging news!

My friend Martyn Norrie sadly died after wrestling with the aftermath of two strokes and hospital infections. Other close friends are wrestling with stroke related issues, and one dear friend has had a relapse of cancer. Three family members and close friends are dealing with the harsh realities of divorce. Nobody plans for these unwanted events, yet they occur every day. They leave physical, emotional and spiritual scars upon our lives, the effects of which are often difficult to reconcile.

So, why do bad things happen to good people, you may ask?

I often hear this question raised in light of irreconcilable suffering, injustice, civil war, illness, violent abuse or fraud. It's my contention that the question of why bad things happen to good people is unhelpful and misleading. Suffering is part of life, and bad things happen to all of us. Good theology supports this, regular conversations with everyday people highlight it, and my craft dictates that I examine it more closely, looking at it from a Christo-centric perspective. That simply means a Christ-centred theological framework. I trust this will be helpful and robust, whether you subscribe allegiance to the Christian faith or not.

One of Jesus's disciples tells us in Luke 18:13 that only God is good. The apostle Paul goes further, informing us in Romans 3:12 that there is no one who does good, as does King David in Psalm 14:3. For some reason there is a misconception held by some, that Christians are good people and consequently safe from unwanted harm or misfortune. Nothing could be further from the truth.

In Mark 10:17-22, Jesus appears to deny His own goodness

in order to highlight humanity's lack. I don't believe there is any conflict here with the biblical imperatives to do good to our fellow humans as image bearers of God. Rather, I am simply highlighting human inability to be the source of all goodness. We are all sinners who fall short of God's standards (Romans 3:23). Furthermore, we are all subject to the laws of a fallen world where war and flood affect the just and the unjust alike (Matthew 5:45). Humans can never claim to match the holiness and goodness of God, His ability to create and sustain life, or to orchestrate believer's salvation made possible through the sacrificial grace of our Lord Jesus Christ on the cross.

Therefore, I find it more helpful to explore *why* God allows bad things to happen; and even more helpful to lift the lid on constructive ways to respond to the suffering we all experience in life. This thought process has helped me fashion responses to my accident, and journey more closely alongside others who are wrestling with their own struggles. Jesus states in John 16:33a that in this world we will always have trouble. Author and Christian apologist C.S. Lewis put it succinctly when he said, "Try to exclude the possibility of suffering which the order of nature and the existence of free wills involved, and you find that you have excluded life itself."[4]

This is largely due to the brokenness of humanity, to sin and the choices we ourselves make (see Romans 5:12, 1 Corinthians 15:21). That said, let me also be very clear that I don't believe suffering is God's way of punishing us, as Job's closest friends thought. It is not in God's nature to follow closely behind us, waiting for us to do wrong so that He can punish us by bringing troubles upon us. It's my conviction that He is far too compassionate and forgiving to treat us in that way.

It follows that we can evaluate our suffering with a sense

of hope and purpose, as I have learnt in my own journey. Furthermore, we may draw on the grace of God which He readily offers to sustain us in our suffering and frailty:

> *But He said to me: My grace is sufficient for you, for My power is made perfect in your weakness.* (2 Corinthians 12:9)

In God's scheme of things, it is possible to be strong even though we feel weak. Can you imagine a winning athlete or a successful businessperson touting their victories in that light? It is countercultural to what we know. This is the nature of what is sometimes referred to as the upside-down kingdom of God. It seems to defy logic, yet God makes it possible if we are willing to trust in His purposes, particularly during hard times.

In the end, I believe God is a willing partner with us in life, offering us the choice to embrace suffering and discover helpful ways of navigating troubled waters instead of avoiding them. My counsellor's advice at the spinal unit comes to mind: "Timothy; you don't have to accept what's happened, but you do have to adapt."

I've reflected on this significantly over the years, although it's taken some time to reconcile in my own mind, to be honest. Accepting my accident raises the question of "Why?", which I could never accommodate or reason through satisfactorily. In fact, most of us will struggle to find a suitable answer to the tough things we will inevitably experience. In other words, human reason will always fall short when it comes to interpreting life's most complex and difficult calamities. (I'm not discounting my own responsibility; for being the one in control of my mountain bike on the day when I fell, with such serious consequences.)

If we choose not to adapt to the 'new norm', then we only make life hard for ourselves and those closest to us. As Holocaust survivor Viktor Frankl wrote: "Everything can be taken from a man but one thing: the last of the human freedoms – to choose one's attitude in any given set of circumstances, to choose one's own way."[5]

I'm determined not to dig a hole for myself. There are still plenty of good reasons to get up in the morning, not the least of which is leaving a legacy of substance and hope for our children and grandchildren. Part of a redemptive attitude and choice is simply being a good neighbour to others, practising generosity and hospitality where opportunity presents itself, and ensuring that my story endures beyond the tangible things of life. As Tony Quinn, motor racing enthusiast and entrepreneur said, "The most valuable thing that you'll leave your children is your story [not your inheritance.]"[6]

All of us have a God-given choice to make good out of a bad situation and to be a channel of God's favour toward our fellow human beings. Investing in others will always enhance our own sense of wellbeing and shine a ray of hope for those on the receiving end. Put simply, distraction through focus on others presents a fresh perspective on suffering, not only for the recipients, but also for those looking on. Often, others will see the reality of our suffering and want to know how we survive and what gives us hope. That's been true for me. "To live is to suffer, to survive is to find some meaning in the suffering."[7]

One of the blessings of serving as a volunteer chaplain at Rotorua Hospital is being able to lift the spirits of sick people by listening to their stories and articulating that it's not only possible to survive but to push back against some of the debilitating realities of our suffering. Often without my saying a word, patients or staff will describe how much better they feel after simply spending time with me. That privilege in itself sustains my life and hope. "People will forget what you said, people will forget what you did, but people will never forget how you made them feel." (Maya Angelou)[8]

Don't get me wrong – I have tough days like the rest of us. I'm careful never to exalt myself or make comparisons with others' grief and suffering, despite some saying that their challenges are minor in contrast to mine. Comparisons are unhelpful. I believe God sees all our suffering as worthy of His equal attention. Yet there are ways of tackling life's challenges head on.

From a strategic perspective, I find it helpful to focus my energies and thoughts on one day at a time. This doesn't come easily for me – I'm a long-term big-picture thinker! By contrast, my wife's philosophy is: "I just do today." She is onto something! After all, God only gives us 24 hours to be concerned about. Each day has enough trouble of its own, as Matthew 6:25-34 tells us. The good news is that Jesus Christ Himself chose to identify with all our suffering, experiencing His own pain on the cross, and returning from the dead to walk alongside us in our journey of faith.

And since we are His children, we are His heirs. In fact, together with Christ, we are heirs of God's glory. But if we are to share His glory, we must also share His suffering. (Romans 8:17, NLT)

On the face of it, this sharing in the suffering of Christ that the apostle Paul articulated around 2,000 years ago may seem like bad news. However, the heart of the Christian gospel (which means 'good news') is to bring hope out of our suffering for all those who have faith in the one who shares it, the saviour Jesus Christ (see Romans 10:9-10, Ephesians 2:8-9).

While there are some commonalities amongst different faith systems, there is no other world religion, philosophy or belief that is unique in this regard: teaching that a divine being reaches down to our level and invites us to share in His journey, both in this world and beyond. In his book *Romans Unplugged*, Les Brighton wrote:

> *But the God who is our eyes and ears and hearts invites us to join Him where He already is, in the nakedness of need, in the heart of the struggle. He gives us a share in what He is already doing in the world. In its understanding of suffering, Christianity is unique among the religions. Buddhism seeks above all things to avoid it. Judaism and Islam see it as a threat of judgement or perhaps tragedy, which ultimately comes from God. Hinduism sees it as a consequence of sins committed in a previous life, but also as a power within the world, to be placated or even celebrated. ... It is no mistake that the symbol of Christianity is a cross. Just as suffering is at the heart of the mystery of the world, so the way God takes personal responsibility for it is at the heart of the good news.*[9]

It's my belief that, in Jesus Christ, God chose to be present here in this world, to embrace suffering in its entirety, and to carry the weight of all our wrongdoing on the cross – the place where forgiveness is wrought on our behalf. Though it is not easy to comprehend, Jesus is both fully human and fully divine. He chose to walk in our shoes, to love human beings through word and action, but also to obey God through sacrificing His own life on our behalf.

Whatever else our pain entails, we are not cosmically alone in it, and so our pain is not futile, but now or meaningless if we will open ourselves to the possibility of a living, loving, suffering God.[10]

In fact, becoming part of God's family means we take on the responsibility of giving up our own lives in sacrifice for others (Luke 8:21). We enter into their pain to ensure they don't feel alone, to partner with God, to live, love and suffer alongside the broken-hearted, the lost and the lonely. By doing so, we embrace the heart of God's Church, the *ecclesia*, to be a restorative force in a world of need.

Perhaps the most powerful example is the apostle Paul in the New Testament (Acts 9:1-19). After a miraculous encounter with God, he finds a new calling, turning full circle from his mission to oppress Jesus' followers and choosing to love them instead, even to reach people from other cultures, entering into their suffering and following the example of Christ whom he served. It was a costly journey, as verse 16 of the text says, "I will show him how much he must suffer for my name." But it was also a fulfilling journey as God gave him the strength to endure it.

And I thank Christ Jesus our Lord who has enabled me, because he counted me faithful, putting me into the ministry. (1 Timothy 1:12, NKJV)

Rebecca MacLachlan posed the question: "How could a loving God allow so much suffering?"[11]

Of course, I could blame God for not alleviating my suffering, forgetting that my freedom is the very reason He chooses not to intervene. If He did, I may likely accuse Him of being a controlling God, so He can't win! In fact, He has too much integrity to lie or go against His own written words and promises, just as the biblical narrative demonstrates.

> *God is not a man, so He does not lie. He is not human, so He does not change His mind. Has He ever spoken and failed to act? Has He ever promised and not carried it through?* (Numbers 23:19, NLT)

> *So, God has given both His promise and His oath. These two things are unchangeable because it is impossible for God to lie. Therefore, we who have fled to Him for refuge can have great confidence as we hold to the hope that lies before us.* (Hebrews 6:18, NLT)

God doesn't have to explain Himself. Our understanding of His actions is always going to be limited because we simply aren't God! In fact, since the time of Adam and Eve we will continue to let Him down as humans, not to mention the very people with whom He created us to be in relationship.

If we choose to accept God's gift of salvation and embark on an intimate and personal journey with Jesus Christ, then suffering takes on a new significance:

> *But if you suffer for doing good and you endure it, this is commendable before God. To this you were called, because Christ suffered for you, leaving you an example that you should follow in His steps.* (1 Peter 2:20b-21)

In terms of my own journey, I find solace in knowing that

Christians worldwide are experiencing incomprehensible suffering. In fact, I believe that our common belief and trust in God strengthens us in the fight against the schemes of the devil as well.

> *Resist him, standing firm in the faith, because you know that the family of believers throughout the world is undergoing the same kind of sufferings.* (1 Peter 5:9; see also Proverbs 3:5-6, Philippians 4:19)

I'm always inspired by fellow Kiwis who fight back in the face of adversity. Psychologist Lucy Hone is a survivor of the Christchurch earthquakes in 2010 and 2011. A few years later, she experienced the kind of aftershock that no parent wishes for when her 12-year-old daughter was killed in a car crash. Her main survival mechanism is to build resilience in the journey of grief.

> *Throwing yourselves into recovery doesn't mean hiding from grief, pain, misery, aching... If you want to win this fight, you've got to step up and take control... Adopting a philosophy that suffering and death are very much part of life acted as a cornerstone of my grief... Accept that you can (and will) adapt to this loss; that although it may require intentional effort on your behalf, it is utterly possible. Above all, you are not alone.*[12]

In reference to Dr Jared Noel's story, mentioned earlier in Chapter 3, his main survival strategy was to see a peaceful purpose in his journey of suffering, as articulated on his deathbed.

> *I have come to a place of acceptance in these things and so I*

continue to trust... I want to forget that whatever suffering this world serves up as an indiscriminate force that chooses no one in particular, but is as arbitrary as the direction of the wind... I took issue on the basis that life is what it is, and that essentially life is more dynamic when we engage the peaks and the troughs and acknowledge the realities of our world, including its sufferings, and incorporate all of our experiences into how we create meaning. My life took an unexpected detour, not a turn for the worse... Suddenly doors opened up to share my story in ways I had never considered... What I've discovered is that the purpose is in the journey, no matter where that journey leads us... This is why I'm an antihero. I don't talk about conquering, overcoming or being the victor. I talk about the reality of suffering in my life and why I'm at peace with that.[13]

A little closer to home, local identity and running coach Kerry Suter had a mountain bike accident and sustained a spinal injury similar to mine, when his partner Ali was pregnant with their first child. In an interview with TV1, Kerry offered a hopeful and optimistic perspective on life after trauma. "We can't spend our whole time looking over our shoulder. The rainbow's actually always in front of us."[14] He echoes the words of theologian and philosopher Søren Kierkegaard (1843), who said, "Life can only be understood backwards; but it must be lived forwards."[15]

The best way for me to understand Kerry's words is to picture the view in the rear vision mirror of a car. The view reminds us of a road travelled, yet we must maintain a forward focus in order to navigate the road ahead safely. Turn the corner, and we may discover not only a rainbow, but a fertile valley, a snowcapped mountain, an inviting lake on a summer's day, a lonely hitchhiker or the last hopeful kilometres before we reach our destination.

In each of the above examples we see a common thread of human resilience in the face of suffering and grief. My journey into suffering challenges me to trust God and view His kindness towards my family and me, both in the rear vision mirror and on the road ahead. I believe that God is always doing the right thing by us, although we may not see it until after the event!

Does this come easily for me? Absolutely not! I'm human, and I'm not always clear about God's purposes, yet I'm assured that He still cares for me, even on the days when I doubt Him. I find comfort in the words of Job from the Old Testament:

You gave me life and showed me kindness, and in Your providence watched over my spirit. (Job 10:12)

Who could imagine the depth of pain that Job must have experienced, having lost his family in a fire, falling on hard times in his farm business, and enduring leprous skin ulcers all over his body? As noted by author Shane Clifton, theologian Neil Ormerod succinctly echoes the words of Job: "Providence can only be recognized looking backwards, with the eyes of faith; seeing the care of God in the midst of suffering."[16]

Job's understanding of the God who sustains him and keeps him safe is echoed in the Māori concept of manaakitanga – hospitality, kindness, generosity, protection, care and respect. Of course, just as God sustains us, we should practise manaakitanga with others!

This fits with the interpretation of the Hebrew word for

providence – *pequddah*[17] – which inspires and encourages me. In essence, this translates to the mustering of God's oversight, care, and resources. In other words, like any good shepherd, He is the one charged to look after us, equipped to provide for us, present to avail Himself for us, and willing to act on our behalf. Who wouldn't want that?

Furthermore, the prophet Isaiah confirms that God is well qualified to enter into our messy lives and travel the journey with us.

> *He was despised and rejected by men; a man of sorrows and acquainted with our grief.* (Isaiah 53:3, NKJV)

I see another reason why God has allowed my suffering. We are not puppets on a string, but God gives us an avenue to connect with Him through prayer and meditation. It's as if God gives us prayer muscles if we choose to believe in Him, and we need to exercise those muscles in order to maintain fitness in the faith. Technically I shouldn't be alive, given the trauma to my head. After initial surgeries and the second attempt to bring me out of an induced coma, I came to and eventually breathed on my own during my 40 days and nights in ICU. I know people prayed for me, and I will be eternally grateful for that. The Bible commentator F.B. Meyer, in reflecting on his struggles, said, "The greatest tragedy of life is not unanswered prayer but unoffered prayer."[18]

From a Christian perspective, prayer is a spiritual discipline, not for us to feel guilty about when we don't pray enough, but to engage with as those responsible to God for managing and caring for this Earth.

Then God said, let Us make mankind in Our image, in Our likeness; so that they may rule over the fish in the sea and the birds in the sky, over the livestock and all the wild animals, and over all the creatures that move along the ground. (Genesis 1:26)

Therefore, when praying, I must always give thanks, knowing that God is accomplishing His purposes through the power and intercession of His Spirit, even when it feels like He is not listening or is somewhat distant from the field I'm playing on (see Romans 8:26, 12:12, Ephesians 6:18, 1 Thessalonians 5:16-18 and James 5:16). I guess that is the nature of having faith in God, especially during the darkest times of my life.

Former all-star baseball pitcher Dave Dravecky struggled with cancer and eventually lost his arm to the disease. He said this:

I have learned that the wilderness is part of the landscape of faith, and every bit as essential as the mountaintop. On the mountaintop we are overwhelmed by God's presence. In the wilderness we are overwhelmed by His absence. Both places should bring us to our knees, the one in utter awe; the other in utter dependence.[19]

Depending on God in suffering doesn't mean relinquishing our humanity; rather, acknowledging that He partners with us and gives us the capacity to thrive in the midst of difficulty. Though it is hard to comprehend, the same power that raised Jesus from the dead is available to us.

That I might know Him and the power of His resurrection

and may share His sufferings becoming like Him in His death. (Philippians 3:10, ESV. See also Ephesians 1:18-20, John 16:33)

I'm well aware that I couldn't achieve the things I do without God's strength and equipping. Physical, mental and spiritual exhaustion are still real factors for me; on the other hand, I like being physically exhausted at the end of the day because it helps me sleep better at night!

So, can God bring good out of a bad situation – absolutely! In fact, He assures us of hope and promise on the horizon (see Jeremiah 29:11, Romans 5:5, 8:28). The story of Job continues to inspire me in this regard. God didn't take away Job's struggles. He parted the clouds and gave him the ability to see beyond them. I believe He desires to do the same for each of us when going through suffering.

My flesh may be destroyed, yet from this body I will see God. Yes, I will see Him for myself, and I long for that moment. (Job 19:26-27, CEV)

Wherever you are in your journey with God, or even if you question whether a loving God exists, I hope that you can find the courage and faith to reach out and grab the hand of Christ. I can honestly say that He's never let me down. Knowing that He identifies with my suffering gives me hope for the future. My losses are real and my weaknesses are ever present in the shadow of that grief. Even my faith in Jesus doesn't promise me a life free of pain and grief, but it does offer me purpose and hope. God's given me fresh opportunities to make a difference for others, and the endurance to fight another day. I trust He will do the same for you.

> *The dance of life finds its beginnings in grief... Here a completely new way of living is revealed. It is the way in which pain can be embraced, not out of a desire to suffer, but in the knowledge that something new will be born in the pain.* (Henri Nouwen)[20]

Questions for reflection:

What strategies do you employ to tackle the difficult challenges that life brings?

How could you turn your grief around and make good of it for the benefit of others?

How might your suffering look different in the light of God's willingness to suffer for you?

Take a look in the rearview mirror. How does the possibility that God has been carrying you without you knowing it change your perspective on the past?

Consider that your trials are not a full stop, but rather a comma in the journey of life. How might the horizon look different now if you were to trust in God's purposes for the future?

Chapter 7

I'm Broken, But Can I Help You?

God uses broken things. It takes broken soil to produce a crop, broken clouds to give rain, broken grains to give bread, broken bread to give strength.
– Vance Havner, American evangelist and author (1901-1986)[1]

When life changes, with unexpected and tragic outcomes, there is always potential for us to limit the scope of opportunity in our new world, at least in our own minds. I'm not denying that my limited physical function dramatically impacts my life, compared with the way it used to be. I'm broken, and it leaves me frustratingly unable to achieve a lot of things, not the least of which is being able to drive or do simple tasks like scratch my itchy neck! I tell my support workers that scratching my itches is the most important thing they do on their shifts with me, and that's why they get paid the big bucks!

ACC assessed me as having lost 92 percent of all function. That's a massive amount to get your head around! My body gets fatigued, and I have a little bit of old-age memory loss to throw in. However, I still have sound cognitive function and the ability to empathise with the world around me. Surely, I can still be fruitful, whether it be for family, or anyone who just needs somebody to travel the journey alongside them? Jesus's words seem apt:

> Very truly I tell you. Unless a grain of wheat falls into the earth and dies, it remains just a single grain; but if it dies, it bears much fruit. (John 12:24, NRSV)

For example, I have an annual request to speak to the international students at Capernwray Bible School near Cambridge. Students come from Canada, the USA, European countries, and Australia, to name a few. They are often in their gap year before university, exploring options for study and travel. I have learned that they are considering the bigger picture of their purpose in life, where to use their God-given gifts effectively, and how to understand our complex world with its unique cultural, social, theological and philosophical nuances.

I speak to them on the last day of their course, not as an expert, but as someone with some training and a unique story to share. They already have their own life experience, wrestling with what it means to suffer and grieve as broken people within their own world. I love the interactive nature of our time together, as I help them see life through a theological lens. I come away fulfilled and blessed to have spent time with them.

At the other end of the spectrum, we have a lovely, elderly friend called Diane Edwards who lives on her own around the corner from us. Her nearest family live out of town and abroad. We have become close over the years. Recently, she has been experiencing technical issues with her car, which have not been easy to diagnose and resolve. Despite not being able to put a spanner on her vehicle myself, I've been able to converse with her local auto electrician and explain the outcomes in more simple terms, so that she understands the process and feels at ease. I happily stop what I'm doing to make time for her. She is very special; a humble prayer warrior, valued friend and neighbour.

On the family front, I was blessed to participate in our older son's wedding on Saturday 24 November 2018 when Hamish married his sweetheart Jess (née Hansen). They asked me and a friend, Amy Davidson, to share in taking the ceremony (picture 9). Amy led them through the vows, and I encouraged the couple with a specific message for them. I've taken two other weddings with colleagues, but the majority have been on my own.

Hamish and Jess live across town now, along with our dear little grandson Christopher. We are especially grateful to God, given that Christopher was born nine weeks early by caesarean section on 16 August 2021. As I was in my fifties when Christopher was born, I figured that I was way too young to be a grandad, but let me tell you, I'm relishing this new season of life in which Jenny and I find ourselves, able to observe his milestones and character development!

Christopher spent his first few weeks in Waikato Hospital. As a parent or grandparent, it's normal to feel helpless in a situation like this. Even more so for me, as I wasn't able to meet some of the new family's practical needs like mowing the lawns or tidying up around their Rotorua property while they were away. It's an endless frustration for me, not being able to help with their property maintenance, building alterations and the like. However, I could at least join Jenny to pray and support them from a distance, just as many of our family and friends did during this time.

The first time we could see him face-to-face was when he came back to Rotorua Hospital on 7 October (two weeks before his scheduled birth date), where he spent a few weeks before coming home. Six months later, he was putting on weight, feeding well and growing just like a normal little baby. Despite the limited use of my arms, I could manage to feed him a bottle while resting him on my lap in the wheelchair. He came for a few rides in those early days, slept on my lap in church, and performed smiles for grandad whilst lying on a pillow!

On one occasion we ventured to Taylor's Reserve at Papamoa Beach to celebrate Hamish's birthday with fish and chips in front of the sand dunes before they set off to the South Island for a week's holiday. Hamish put Christopher on my lap and secured him to the wheelchair with my scarf. I took off around the park, leaving family in the distance and enjoying precious minutes with Christopher to myself. He hung his left arm over the side as if travelling in a car with his arm out the window (picture 10a)!

Another memorable time for me was visiting the annual Fieldays at Mystery Creek, Hamilton. I used to attend this event in my younger days when working as a mechanic. On this occasion, I travelled with Hamish, Jess, and Christopher. Christopher hopped on my lap while we made our way around the different displays together. There were a couple of times when we took off on our own, leaving Hamish and Jess to have some valuable one-on-one time looking at sites and displays of specific interest to them. They are busy young parents, giving generously of themselves to so many others: family, friends, neighbours and fellow parishioners. So this was a priceless, although brief, time alone. I relished this time with Christopher as his grandad. As you can imagine, the stimulating environment tired him out, and he eventually fell asleep on my lap (picture 10b) when it was almost time to leave.

More recently, Jenny and I were able to attend our first official function as grandparents, sharing afternoon tea with staff and families at Christopher's daycare. It seems you can't avoid attracting the attention of innocent preschoolers when you're in a strange contraption on wheels. Christopher hopped on my lap, and I made my way around the outdoor playground with a string of children in tow. Over the course of an hour or so, I was able to encourage many smiles out of those young children, much to the delight of staff watching on! It was a very fulfilling time, reinforcing that I could help and make a difference in that context, despite my disability.

Family is a sustaining factor for me. We are blessed to still have Callum under our roof and to journey with him as an adult. Aside from our Thursday afternoons together, I'm able to encourage him with the daily challenges he wrestles with, and together with Jenny, celebrate his achievements. Recently, he began a part-time job as park attendant at the local Paradise Valley Animal Park. He has been faithful to the task and loves working with the animals, finding a vocational niche that he enjoys.

Callum is a wonderful uncle to Christopher and is taking this new role in his stride. We take time and opportunities as they arise to speak into his life and learn from him along the way. He is refreshingly open, and honest to a fault. I don't have to go digging for information, as he shares willingly from the heart. Occasionally, he is thrust into looking after me, moving down to our guestroom overnight, and interrupting routines to help me. I've observed that he is very patient and I enjoy proud moments when others speak of his generosity and fortitude.

Despite feeling like a big part of my life has gone through a death experience, I'm enriched to be travelling the road with family, friends, colleagues and members of our community. I know that God's purposes for me remain strong. That dream I had as an 18-year-old to follow God's calling and embark on working with people in a full-time pastoral capacity came to pass at the right time. I've enjoyed senior leadership roles in several churches over the last 28 years. Now, God's call on my life is just as strong although it has a different focus in ministry and community service now.

As the years have gone by, I've been presented with many new and interesting opportunities to extend care and kindness to others in need, to 'pay it forward' as the saying goes. An example of this is being involved in a mentoring programme for others who are new to wheelchair use, either due to sustaining a spinal injury or a medical condition or incident such as a stroke.

This programme was set up by Debbie Wilson, the former owner of our local wheelchair repair company, Seating to Go. Debbie is an occupational therapist and advocate for those who find their mobility has been severely restricted. She is a warm and engaging person, and her whole demeanour really shows how much she cares for her clients.

In 2019, Debbie asked me if I would consider becoming a mentor for the programme, which is usually run over two days or sessions. To begin with, several occupational therapists and support staff set up a local hall or community facility with cones and a range of obstacles. The mentors come alongside participants and encourage them to have a go, coaching them in how to navigate the obstacles. They usually bring along their closest family members and any support workers recruited to care for them during this new season of life.

For my first time mentoring in the project, I was given a pre-teen boy to support. He was non-verbal, but responded warmly to my encouragement, particularly when I demonstrated how to tackle the course.

After work in the hall, depending on the weather, we go outside to the streets, navigating the nearby terrain, up and down kerbs and so on. In some cases, we visit individuals in their home and help them navigate their surroundings. It's an absolute privilege to identify with and help those on similar journeys to mine, equipping them to progress with confidence in the early stages of adjusting to life on wheels. About 2,400 years ago, the great philosopher Aristotle put it succinctly: "What is the essence of life? To serve others and to do good."

In April 2021, I was asked if I could fill in for someone at one of Debbie's programmes in Hamilton. I wasn't overly enthusiastic about going, partly because of the travel involved, but also because it was cold and wintry. I just wanted to stay at home in the warmth and work on other things in my office. However, it did present an opportunity to visit my brother Steve, so I decided to go.

I was assigned a 70-year-old woman called Edna who had recently had a stroke. We worked through the session as instructed by the occupational therapists. The second session required me to visit the retirement home where she lived. Edna had just acquired an electric wheelchair two weeks earlier, so it was all fresh for her, and that day she had her daughter and husband in tow.

It was quite hard work helping Edna, as I discovered whilst guiding her around the gardens and footpaths of the complex. The stroke had left one side of her body lacking important function for daily use. As a result, she kept veering left towards the inner garden wall and a drop to a manicured piece of lawn. It was the equivalent of a couple of steps down, so there was a risk of her falling over and further injuring herself! Nonetheless, Edna was keen to learn, despite her physical ailments.

I felt some emotion welling up inside as we concluded our time together. She said, "Tim, I feel a whole lot more confident," and thanked me for my patience with her. I reflected to Jenny later that it had definitely been right to go. It made a difference for her and was fulfilling for me as a mentor.

While I've alluded to it before, allow me to touch on matters of healing and wellbeing. Our bodies already have an amazing God-given capacity to heal, whether from a scratch or orthopaedic surgery. In the case of spinal cord injury, there are advances in stem cell replacement and neural regeneration. In the early stages of my recovery, the physiotherapists were using findings from studies in neuroplasticity which show that the brain can regenerate neural pathways and therefore benefits from a combination of thought processes and physical stimulation. Gains can be made in the first two years after the injury.

This was true for me in terms of physical function and muscle movement. After those first two years, though, progress has been fairly static, which is often the case for patients with incomplete spinal injuries. The latest research literature drawn from more than 5,000 publishers gives hope for people with physical and neural impairments such as mine. In an article published by American Society of Interventional Pain Physicians, reviewers concluded that: "Using [stem cells from human bone marrow] can help stimulate healing, and neural regeneration remains a tantalizing possibility."[2]

I'm not so naïve as to disregard 21st century advances in healing through modern medicine. For me, that's evidence enough that humans have been equipped with a unique and innate God-given ability to make advances that benefit our health.

The Christian worldview for the beginning of life acknowledges the input of a creative and intelligent God, in contrast to the idea that life may have randomly emerged from pond scum or a Big Bang, as some believe. With all due respect for our different beliefs about the source of human life, we all grow and have to deal with the frailties of our humanity, with minds and bodies that let us down with multiple sclerosis and cancer, or with anything that affects our vocational and recreational pathways in detrimental ways.

Still, I believe it remains God's prerogative to heal – through modern medicine, or by miraculous means as He did in Bible times, or through a combination of both. I'm a product of the latter, when you consider my level of injury, the risk of infection at the time, and comments from the physicians who saw me and articulated that my life was in the balance. In theory, I shouldn't be able to string enough words together to form a cohesive sentence, let alone write a book! This is due to taking a direct hit on my frontal lobes, which is where we plan, organise, concentrate and solve problems.

I am alive, however, with this broken body and my mind intact. This is how we explain my physiology to our grandson. I believe my ability to function as much as I am able, is due to the providence of God and to the prayers of many who earnestly interceded, by faith, on my behalf. All I can say is that I'm humbled and enormously grateful.

For example, I have to use my intercostal muscles when breathing and speaking publicly, as normal diaphragm function is somewhat compromised. Yet, despite the extra effort involved in projecting my voice, I can still share my story. How is this possible? I can only conclude that the 'man upstairs' is on my case. I'm assured that God is ready and waiting for each one of us to reach out and trust Him with our lives, especially the difficult things that are both puzzling and mysterious to us in the bigger picture. He may not give us the answers we want or act when we want Him to, but at least I believe He is listening when we pray! It's often not until after the event that we realise He's been at work on our behalf. That's been true for me despite not being fully functional.

I believe absolutely that miraculous healing is a sovereign work of God that is still relevant today. Many people believe physical healing to be the focus of the prophet Isaiah's words in the Old Testament:

> *But He was wounded for our transgressions, crushed for our iniquities; upon Him was the punishment that made us whole, and by His bruises we are healed.* (Isaiah 53:5, NRSV)

However, it's important to note that the broader healing of which Isaiah speaks, translates to a spiritual healing from the sickness of our sin that separates us from God.

In other words, we are brought into a place of healing with God because Jesus Christ saved us from the punishment we deserved for our wrongdoing. That's the essence of the Christian gospel, a provision of God's grace toward the world He loves and with whom He desires to be in relationship. That grace provides peace if, by faith, we accept God's gift of salvation through Christ. What follows, I believe, is a lifetime of healing which God provides for His children who constantly fall short of His standards because we are still fallen creatures with broken bodies and minds.

Thus, the wellbeing we so desperately crave in life is appropriated through humble faith in the God above. One commentator offers a helpful thought in this regard: "It was our peace, or what is more in accordance with the full idea of the word, our general wellbeing, our blessedness, which these sufferings arrived at and secured."[3]

I do not subscribe to a prosperity doctrine which interprets the words of Isaiah as offering physical healing for all time if we simply name and claim it. That said, I do believe that through prayer we have the confidence that God is always listening and wanting to respond in line with His purposes, if we call on Him in faith. He may even surprise us in ways we hadn't imagined or anticipated, simply because He is a gracious God.

> *And this is the boldness we have in Him, that if we ask anything according to His will, He hears us.* (1 John 5:14, NRSV)

My healing remains a work of God's grace at His discretion, whether it be here on Earth or in heaven. I would love to walk and run again; relieve my wife of daily tasks like doing the dishes and taking the car for a warrant of fitness; do repair work on my son and daughter-in-law's house; hug my grandson; rub my wife's back; or attend to maintenance on our property – the list goes on.

Thinking about these losses – from which there is no coming back – creates an ongoing tension and a constant ache in the core of my heart. Shonagh Walker and Sara Mulcahy note that, "Loss affects us all and is one of the most traumatic life events." They quote grief counsellor Wendy Liu:

> *All of us experience some level of loss throughout our lifetimes. These include the breakdown of a relationship, miscarriage, death, divorce, the loss of a pet, losses through changes in the workplace, loss of sexual intimacy, or loss of independence through illness or injury.*[4]

I cannot demand healing, otherwise I might feel guilty, as if my faith is second-rate, or that my prayers are not substantial enough, because I still have tetraplegia at the end of the day. For the sake of my wife and myself, and indeed for our wider family, friends and community, I need to live well-grounded in each day that is before us, lest we go crazy in pursuit of a distant reality. In other words, God may want us to have a broader understanding of healing and wellbeing than just my physical condition.

I see no contradiction between suffering and healing; rather, I should hold these in tension and celebrate what I'm able to achieve in God's strength despite my limitations. From a biblical perspective, there are other tensions to live with, such as between grace and truth, or between God's sovereignty and human responsibility.

I feel an obligation towards others as a servant of God, who is the custodian of the environment in which each of us lives. We can enhance life for the people we rub shoulders with every day, or suck it dry from them in mindless fashion. The implication is that we ourselves need to be in a space of relative wellbeing, which we can find in part by helping our fellow human beings.

Australian author, ethicist and theologian Shane Clifton sustained a spinal injury in the same year as me, also through a bike accident. In a paper titled 'The Dark Side of Healing', he writes:

> *Our goal isn't impossible perfection, or perfect health, but rather to tell a meaningful story or be part of a meaningful story. We can flourish, even though sometimes we suffer, if our lives are invested with meaning. ... For most people with long-term disabilities, however, coming to accept that situation, to*

learn to live and even flourish with it, is one of the essential stages of healing. This suggests a potential way forward, a broadening of what is intended by the affirmation of divine healing, redirected to what I shall call "wellbeing".[5]

One example of investing my life with meaning was when I commenced my regular Friday morning ward round as a volunteer chaplain at Rotorua Hospital one day in early December 2023. I entered the expansion room in the orthopaedic ward which provides extra bed space for patients when nursing staff and funding allows it.

There was only one bed there, which was being made up by a nurse trainee. She was clearly new, as she wasn't even wearing the appropriate uniform. I soon found out that she was fully trained in her native country of India but had yet to complete the requirements for working as a registered nurse in New Zealand.

As we engaged in conversation, I learnt that her husband and child remained in India, and that she was trying to gain employment and a foot in the door of our country, so that the family could join her here. As I asked about her life and family, she stepped aside from the bed for a moment and her eyes moistened as she paused to contain her emotions. My own tears were beginning to well up at this point. I guess I'm just a big softy at heart!

I backed off and apologised, saying that I hadn't intended to upset her. She said that wasn't the case – she appreciated my questioning and my care and empathy for her plight. We chatted for a little while longer (I'm always mindful that staff have a job to do, and I respect their time). I sensed that she might appreciate a word of prayer, which is something I offer if I discern that it is appropriate and warranted. She thanked me and I went on my way.

My time talking with the nurse from India was, for me, a meaningful encounter, even if it was only for 15 minutes. Engaging with others like this allows me to flourish and boosts my wellbeing; the discipline of service acts as a means of healing in my life. I consider this to be achieving a broader appropriation of the work of Christ on the cross.

Russian novelist and Nobel Peace Prize winner Leo Tolstoy, probably best known for his book *War and Peace* (1869), stated that: "Only people who are capable of loving strongly can also suffer great sorrow, but this same necessity of loving serves to counteract their grief and heals them."[6]

With that broader understanding of healing in mind, I am determined to love and encourage those whom God brings across my pathway, assured that He will sustain me whatever the cost. As psychologist and Auschwitz survivor, Viktor Frankl, wrote,

> *The way in which a person accepts their fate and all the suffering it entails, the way in which they take up the cross, gives them ample opportunity – even under the most difficult circumstances – to add a deeper meaning to their life.*[7]

In conclusion, to take up the cross is to identify with the sufferings of Christ and love the people of our world until it hurts, knowing that our pain and sorrow is worth the cost of bringing hope to their horizons. To paraphrase John's gospel: No greater love is there than laying down your life for others (John 15:13). That's why we can say with absolute conviction that Jesus is hope personified.

As a follower of Christ, I feel a responsibility to walk in His footsteps in as much as He gives me the energy to fulfil that journey. If I was still working as a mechanic when I had my accident, there'd be no option of continuing that career path. However, I'm convinced that God has still given me a reason to live, a platform from which to tell my story, and a part to play in this community and beyond. Life is still worth living, despite being broken, despite the ever-present frustration and grief. I'm going to give it my best for as long as I'm able.

Questions for reflection:

If you were to look beyond the daily struggles or tragic circumstances of your life, who would benefit from your skills and time?

In what ways would you view life differently if God healed you today from your physical or mental impairments? How might you use your newfound freedom to journey with and invest in others who are going through similar experiences?

From where do you draw strength?

What does wellbeing mean for you, holistically? How could that influence those you journey with?

How could you explore the spiritual element of your life that may be at work on your behalf?

Chapter 8

Channels of Hope from the Weary

*We give great honour to those who endure under suffering.
For instance, you know about Job, a man of great endurance.
You can see how the Lord was kind to him at the end,
for the Lord is full of tenderness and mercy.*
(James 5:11, NLT)

In this chapter, I will briefly observe the lives of four local Kiwis from my community whom I admire and identify with. Each has a different story of suffering and trauma which I will explore, looking at its context and the impact on their own lives as well as others'. I will describe their responses and how they keep smiling while channelling hope to others in significant ways. There are common threads in these stories which I trust will inspire and motivate you on your own journey, just as they have done for me.

These individuals each gave me permission to tell their story. Out of respect and for partial anonymity, I will simply state their first names.

Bill's story

Bill is a local identity and fellow parishioner, born on 6 May 1966, making him just 12 days my senior. He grew up in the western suburb of Fordlands, described in 2017 as "the most deprived suburb of Rotorua,"[1] and used as the setting for Alan Duff's bestselling novel *Once Were Warriors* which inspired the 1994 movie of the same name.

The locals call it 'Ford Block', and I must say that I've journeyed over the years with some special people from Ford Block, despite it getting a bad rap in terms of crime and gang presence. We once considered living there in the early stages of my ministry at Rotorua Baptist Church.

Bill has four sisters and two brothers. He describes his late mum as a faith healer who gambled a lot. She died when he was 21 years old, although his dad is still alive. As a young boy, Bill lived on the streets, getting into trouble for sniffing petrol at the age of seven. He got involved with several gangs and ended up in a youth penitentiary at the age of 16.

He wrestled with poor mental health, the treatment drugs worsening his state of mind to the extent that he became suicidal and ended up spending more than 10 years in different mental health facilities. He was sectioned four times to Tokanui Psychiatric Hospital, historically one of New Zealand's largest psychiatric institutions. Despite this rough period of life, he says, "In jail I always knew that Jesus Christ was with me and will continue to be with me." He puts this down to becoming a Christian at the age of nine as a result of a spiritual encounter with God. He simply says that God greeted him. He even baptised a guy in the bathtub at Tokanui!

Bill has weathered those rough years of dysfunction and drug abuse to the point where he's been well enough to engage in different jobs, ranging from tree-felling to picking kiwifruit. He has volunteered at St Vincent de Paul's and continues to work part-time at Mainfreight Rotorua where he's been a valuable employee since 2011.

There are several things I admire about Bill – he has no inhibitions and is generous and caring toward others in our community. He is open about taking medication for epilepsy, although he is independent enough to live on his own. He will turn up to church barefoot and proudly wave a blanket above his head with a picture of Jesus on it, clearly identifying his Saviour and the focus of his worship and faith. Most notable is his singing; it's of no concern to him that he can't sing in tune with fluctuating levels of volume. His worship of God is unrestrained, and he often repeats the words "all the way." He enjoys fellowship at his local church and says. "Knowing God gives me strength and wellbeing, and that is what brings me hope."

His goal is simply that he wants to help wherever he can. Evidence of this is his weekly attendance at a Wednesday morning tea called 'The Cupboard' at St John's Presbyterian Church. I'm privileged to be a chaplain and member of the facilitating team who serve the patrons there from week to week. Families and individuals living in emergency housing, motels, cars, or on the street come along. Bill sees himself as the gatekeeper, often sitting near the front door, keeping an eye on who is coming and going, greeting people, but watching for unacceptable behaviour.

Near the end of January 2023, I greeted him at the end of a Sunday service at the Baptist Church. He'd been to church at St John's that morning and came to the Baptist Church afterwards to thank people who gave him a food parcel at Christmas time. He gave the whole box to his neighbour who had no food at all. How could you not be humbled and inspired by this man?

Rob's story

Rob was working as a physical fitness instructor at the Air Force base in Shelly Bay, Wellington. On 20 April 1980, he was on his way north to compete in the Rotorua Marathon with his first wife Bronwyn and a friend. They lost control of their ute in the wet weather and ended up down a bank south of Taihape. Rob (then aged 27), fell out the window and sustained a spinal injury at T7/8 vertebrae. He had to call out for about 30 minutes before they found him. His dog fell from the back of the utility vehicle at the same time but was later found to be okay.

Damage to nerves in this area generally results in paraplegia. Implications are loss of bowel and bladder control, impairment to abdominal and back muscles, and varying degrees of nerve pain. Rob had a couple of nights in Whanganui Hospital before being flown to Burwood Hospital in Christchurch where he spent only nine weeks in rehab. Rob told Bronwyn that if she wanted to separate and move out, she should do it without delay. She declined the offer.

Beds were in short supply, so they sent him to Wigram Air Base for three weeks. They didn't prepare for his unique needs before he arrived unfortunately, so the accommodation wasn't ideal. Nonetheless, he pressed through, managing with minimal help. A similar thing happened later when he was moved to the Hobsonville Air Force base. People are just not au fait with the unique needs of somebody with a spinal injury, as I know well!

He bought a home in Henderson a year or two later and stayed there for 12 years. During this time, his wife made a trip to Australia, met a man and eventually left Rob to marry him. After that, Rob met Sharon when she was working at the Rehabilitation League in Mount Eden. They married in 1987. Rob describes Sharon as "a remarkable, devoted and protective woman," and I honour her for her faithfulness to Rob over the years.

Rob couldn't continue as a fitness instructor after his accident, so he went on to study occupational therapy and worked at that for 24 years. He helped others with accessibility needs and worked in the area of mental health for two years. He also worked in Māori Health Services, focusing on drug and alcohol rehabilitation. During this time, he coached 8- to 14-year-old students with their unique sporting needs through CCS Mini Olympics, travelling with them throughout the regions for 10 years. He maintained good fitness himself and tackled the Honolulu Marathon in his wheelchair – possibly the first to do so both on foot and on wheels, he believes!

Rob moved to Rotorua in 1995 where he contracted to ACC for two years, working as a team leader arranging assessments for clients with disabilities. I think this is ironic, given his need of ACC assessments himself now! Then he was with Support Net for two years as a team leader doing similar work. Following that, he set up a private practice as an occupational therapist. He loved helping people with their rehab, motivated more by improving their wellbeing than the money he earned in the process!

During this time, he worked for Bay of Plenty (BOP) Rugby as a junior rugby liaison officer, teaching rugby skills to teenagers part-time. He was general manager of Te Whare Hauora O Ngongotahā for 12 years, helping improve the general health and wellbeing of local Māori, with a focus on mental health in particular. He won a volunteer of the year award for services to junior rugby at the BOP sports awards. He served voluntarily at the bowling club where he remains a valued community representative.

In total, Rob worked from 1983 to 2012; that's 29 years of employment – quite a feat when you consider that many people with spinal injuries stop working by choice, depending on their capacity. ACC likes people to work in a paid capacity to some degree if possible. In my experience, ACC has only recently begun recognising voluntary work, in terms of being prepared to fund related needs and provide the necessary support.

Regarding the struggles that affected him one way or another, Rob found that living with a disability was easier than coping with the trauma of a marriage breakdown. He had a lot of urinary tract infections in the early stages, which could have been mitigated by different management methods. He has always been fit and independent. Now, his life is structured so much that it is difficult to be as spontaneous and free as he used to be. Rob has ongoing issues with dysfunctional support agencies and support workers, especially those who don't show initiative and lack sufficient empathy to do their job well.

Rob has been in a wheelchair now for 44 years, but states that the last four and a half years have been the hardest, due to pressure sores, wound infections, and bone health issues which have kept him on bed rest. This takes real patience! His skin is so vulnerable that he suffers setbacks each time he gets up and leaves the house in his wheelchair. Being on bed rest has reduced his quality of life significantly, but he describes it as "my lot for the rest of my life."

He especially misses connections with others, especially through his rugby and sport. He was performing so well at the age of 17 that he was potentially on track to become an All Black. He also finds it difficult not being able to foster relationships in the way he used to.

His current job requires good eyesight for working on his

computer while lying awkwardly in bed. Unfortunately, he is not getting the necessary support and understanding to have his cataracts fixed, and he expresses frustration that this is not being remedied quickly. Rob is generally upbeat and happy to have a laugh, but he's honest about the fact that he can easily mask the tough days by responding with the words: "I'm good." Many of us would identify with this.

I have observed his resilient demeanour shining through in the time I've known him. It is to his credit that he continues to give his time to help others in need, despite living with a debilitating life injury. He is a blessing and inspiration to many in our community and has an important role as a peer supporter for others with spinal injuries in our region.

He admits he has his down days, but looks to the positive, both for himself and others. There's a Chinese proverb that captures this well: "If you want happiness for an hour, take a nap. If you want happiness for a day, go fishing. If you want happiness for a year, inherit a fortune. If you want happiness for a lifetime, help somebody." Rob says, "Leaving a legacy of helping others who are wrestling with difficult life issues is what drives me."

When reflecting on the past, Rob says he used to be fiercely independent and focused on himself, but now he's able to consider the needs of others. He is great at problem-solving and uses that skill to benefit those who may be stuck with the impact of difficult life circumstances. He attributes this skill to being the oldest in his family, although that's not necessarily true for all of us. I see synergy with the words of Lucy Hone, who wrote:

Recent psychological studies have demonstrated that optimism is a key protective mechanism against depressive symptoms in the face of trauma, regardless of individual's culture of origin... optimists focus on solutions when change is possible and use acceptance and humour when it's not. They are also more accurate in their assessment of how much control they have, and less likely to deny and avoid problems... Reivich and Shatte explain how this kind of flexible thinking style relates to resilience. "The most resilient people are those who have cognitive flexibility and can identify all the significant causes of the adversities they face... They are realists and they don't ignore the factors that are permanent or pervasive. Nor do they waste their valuable reserves of resilience ruminating about events or circumstances outside of their control. They channel the problem-solving resources into the factors they can control, and, through incremental change, they begin to overcome, steer through, bounce back and reach out."... Realistic optimism requires maintaining a positive outlook without denying reality, appreciating the positive aspects of any given situation without overlooking the negatives.[2]

Rob is confident enough to fight for his own needs, though, like me, he acknowledges the help that ACC gives. His family of eight siblings is also a great support for Rob, although sometimes they need a gentle reminder to visit their brother when he's stuck in bed! In terms of faith, Rob comes from a Catholic tradition and, while he does not attend church much now, he still holds to a belief in the Creator God, and that heaven and hell are real places. He finds hope and encouragement in trusting that God is always watching over his life.

Rob is a true Kiwi pioneer, punching above his weight and serving sacrificially for the benefit of others. I admire his resilience in the face of insurmountable bodily restraints.

Michelle's story

Michelle had a rocky start to life. She was born 11 weeks early, and when another child in the neonatal unit died, her mother felt guilty that Michelle had survived. Her parents were devout Catholics, but their marriage was very shaky. One of her grandmothers passed away unexpectedly when Michelle was nine months old.

When she was nearly four years old, Michelle came across her younger baby sister who had fallen into the family swimming pool. She had enough sense to alert her mum who called an ambulance. Her sister was resuscitated and survived. Despite her dad trying to help by distracting her, Michelle's experience with her sister's near-death experience at the pool caused her to have anxiety attacks. Then her parents went bankrupt, and the family had to uproot and move to another Bay of Plenty town.

Michelle loved learning at school, despite being a very quiet and introverted child. More trauma occurred when she was six – her grandfather died, and her mother struggled with sickness after having her teeth removed. She describes her mother as having a 'toxic tongue'; she drank a lot, and her mental health deteriorated. Her father also drank to numb the pain of living with his wife's behaviour. This turned him into an aggressive man. Michelle remembers gathering her siblings and finding safe places to hide with them, in fear of their parents. The effects of this kind of atmosphere are described by priest and author Henri Nouwen: "Fear makes us move away from each other to a 'safe' distance or move toward each other to a 'safe' closeness, but fear does not create the space where true intimacy can exist."[3]

Her other grandmother also had health issues. As a result

of her heart condition, she came to live with the family when Michelle was in her early teens. Michelle found her intimidating, which didn't help make her home a very safe place to be.

Despite living in a dysfunctional household, Michelle developed a passion for music, and she learnt to play the keyboard and a range of wind instruments. She joined a choir and loved to sing, which fostered her intimacy with God.

When she was 16, a friend invited her to a local Presbyterian Church. As a result of the church's friendship and gospel message, she became a Christian and joined the music team. She remembers her father saying, "Most girls your age are asking to go to town, when you're asking to go to church." By the time she was 18 years old, her love for music led her to study at Hillsong College in Australia. This involved a variety of topics from creative arts to Christian ethics. She excelled in singing and was given opportunities to direct the choir for Sunday worship. This brought a great deal of joy to her heart. Furthermore, she helped vulnerable families in the local community during her spare time. Her own lived experience gave her a genuine understanding of their unique needs.

> *Your lived experience is a valuable asset that can help you connect with and support others.*[4]

Two years later, Michelle had to drop her studies and move back to New Zealand because her family situation had become dire. Her parents had decided to separate, so Michelle moved to Waikato with her mother. By now, her father was severely depressed, and her mother had begun to exhibit narcissistic behaviour, excessive control and superiority over Michelle and her siblings. She said, "I was holding onto the fairy tale that my parents would stay stable and connected throughout my life." As a result of this, she only knew a distorted idea of conditional love, walking on eggshells and becoming a scapegoat for her siblings, one of whom her mum considered to be the golden child.

By now, Michelle's singing voice had improved to the extent that she could sing for others. Looking back now, though, she considers that she felt the need to perform for people in the hope of winning her parents' love. Feelings of anxiety surfaced again, particularly when she was tired. The overwhelming message in her mind was that she wasn't good enough for her parents. This led to a struggle with anorexia for a couple of years.

Eventually, she went on to study teaching and was offered a pastoral role in a church. The job didn't work out financially, so Michelle found herself working 40 hours at a supermarket checkout in order to survive. Sadly, the church she was involved with went through a split. Michelle says, "I felt another layer of disappointment and mistrust," as memories of her dysfunctional family crept back into her life. This was a challenging season in her faith journey, but she held onto God and wrote a book to record this journey for the benefit of others.

She returned to Australia in 2009, hoping for a fresh start teaching music at Hillsong. However, she experienced further change when she lost this job as a result of the global financial crisis. It was a challenging time as she couldn't find any suitable work. So she applied to Bethlehem Tertiary Institute back in New Zealand to complete her teaching qualifications.

Despite ongoing negativity and things not going to plan with a job application in her hometown, a senior teacher at the interview gave her an affirming word. This teacher has become a treasured friend and an influential figure in her life. Michelle ended up working at a satellite branch of a Christian school, starting with lesser roles until she was given her own class. She remains a valued music teacher at the school and a key member of the music team in a local church. She has grown in confidence and took a year off in 2024 to serve among the homeless and vulnerable people of Los Angeles City, also visiting Uganda to support and witness the famous Watoto Children's Choir.

Looking back, Michelle is glad to have had some help through counselling, although she still wrestles with people-pleasing and the need to feel secure in her own skin. She still has an ongoing propensity for anxiety and says, "Everybody walks with a limp. Just because you're a Christian doesn't mean your life is going to be easy." The biblical accounts in Genesis 32 of Jacob's wrestling injury with the angel, and the apostle Paul's thorn in the flesh in 2 Corinthians 12 come to mind. Nonetheless, going through 'dark valleys', as she describes them, has given her empathy for others, a desire to be authentic, nonjudgmental and encouraging. She's grown a deep understanding and belief that, at the end of the day, God is who He says He is, in contrast to inconsistent and controlling people like her parents.

Michelle sometimes feels that God is distant from her, but she renews that connection through nature and music. When navigating the ups and downs of life, she says, "God is incapable of lying, and He has been with me in my lowest and mundane places, just as much as He is with me in the high places." In response to the question of what gets her out of bed in the morning, she says,

> I recognise that for this time I am planted here on this earth. I'm asking – how can I reflect Christ's love to others and make

an impact for God's glory? My biggest hope is seeing Jesus face to face one day in eternity. I know the author of hope and want to pass that on to other people.

Wow! I see Michelle as an amazing individual, who, in spite of overwhelmingly debilitating circumstances, is offering her gifts in service to others, holding her head up high as a truly resilient Kiwi.

Rob II's story

Rob was born in Te Kōpuru, near Dargaville in Northland. He did a brief stint farming and worked as a government valuer for a few years before following the call into pastoral ministry. After theological training, he worked for nine years as a Baptist pastor before venturing into mission work amongst the poorer cultures of Southeast Asia.

Rob invested further time studying theology in the United States before returning to New Zealand and working for the well-known mission agencies, Tearfund and World Vision. He also lectured at Carey Baptist College during this time. Since retiring, he's held some interim pastorates in Baptist churches and continues to support mission and development work in countries like India (where his daughter and son-in-law are missionaries).

Sadly, Rob went through a messy and painful marriage breakdown and has worked through deep regrets from this difficult period of his life. Furthermore, he was shocked at the age of 77 to be given a diagnosis of cancer. A lump the size of a fist was discovered in his left lung. They said he might only live three to six months if it wasn't removed. He came down with Covid-19 at the same time and had vital surgery for the cancer that same year. He says, "To get through life without a crisis or two is rare."

Rob went through subsequent chemo, radiation and infusions, but was not given full clearance as the cancer resisted treatment. He speaks very positively about oncology staff and the New Zealand hospital system. Not content to wallow in this medical quagmire, he has made good use of the downtime by completing projects he started as a Bible scholar and writer, producing significant and ongoing works of biblical exposition.

His future is uncertain, given that nearly four years later, he still has nodules in both lungs. Despite that, he is a very active chap! He says, "I am breathless whenever I exert myself which I do often with tennis, lawn-mowing and gardening every week. Apart from that, I hardly know I am unwell… I live life as much as I can as long for as I can. I am ready to embrace the next life where there is no pain and suffering."

Rob has remarried and is faithfully supported by his wife Jan. I had the privilege of performing that ceremony myself and continue to witness their vibrant and fruitful partnership. They embrace mutual relationships of love and support, particularly with those in their local church. Rob's greatest hope lies in a firm conviction: "The resurrection is the world's greatest gift. I know Jesus rose again and I believe I shall too. I am ready to die knowing I have lived a very full life and enjoyed it."

Rob is a trooper, not content to retreat and rest but to use every ounce of his energy and skills to serve and inspire for the betterment of our community and beyond!

I can see common threads in the lives of all these people. They are all honest about the reality of life, not discounting their suffering, but finding a way through it with a sense of hope for the future.

Our bodies are buried in brokenness, but they will be raised in glory. They are buried in weakness but will be raised in strength. (1 Corinthians 15:42-43, NLT)

Despite the impact on the lives of these remarkable New Zealanders, and not forgetting those closest to them, they are forging a productive pathway, mentally, physically, spiritually and relationally. In every case they are exhibiting an intentional focus on others which, in turn, is helping them navigate their own difficult pathway.

To me, this echoes the kind of resilience about which Lucy Hone speaks. It encapsulates a positive Kiwi outlook. But, more than that, it is a great example we can adopt and use to further strengthen the fabric of our own lives. I would add a warning that we need to be careful not to copy or compare ourselves with others. As several famous people are believed to have said, "Comparison is the thief of joy."[5]

My advice is to look to your own strengths, embrace your struggles, and find the niche where you can make a difference for others who are struggling. That's what the lives of phenomenal New Zealanders are made of.

My faith enables me to look beyond the suffering I've experienced in life. That's where hope is found, in the God above, who loves each one of us with the same passion that Jesus Christ displayed here on Earth more than 2,000 years ago. That sense of hope is something each one of us so desperately needs to navigate the troubled waters of our time. As the writer to the Hebrews states:

What is faith? It is the confident assurance that what we want is going to happen. It is the certainty, that what we hope

for is waiting for us, even though we cannot see it up ahead.
(Hebrews 11:1, TLB)

Please note that the Hebrews writer is not referring to the wants of this life, but to what the life beyond offers, where I believe suffering and death will be no more, where the kingdom that Jesus began is fulfilled in heaven because He obeyed the Father's will and purpose for His life.

Questions for reflection:

Consider your own plight in the light of the stories above. Which threads do you identify as being part of your story?

How could focusing on others bolster your own life?
What would it take to make that happen?

What does hope mean for you despite your difficult circumstances? How could you begin painting the picture of your horizon in a more colourful and fruitful way? Who could feature in that picture that you hadn't imagined before?

Chapter 9

Sharing the Beauty of 'God's Own'

Hope looks for a better future as well but sees the present as a stepping stone towards that future.
– Graham Leo, Australian writer and educator[1]

Some might consider that being in a wheelchair offers nothing more than a bleak future. I'm here to tell you that despite my limitations, and with the help of others, I can still enjoy some of the most stunning scenery that this beautiful land of Aotearoa has to offer. Allow me to share a couple of special memories and experiences that give further depth to the hope I carry in what's possible. Put your travel shoes on and continue the journey with me, here in 'God's own' country.

It was Wednesday 26 February 2020, a stunning morning in Westland's Tai Poutini National Park on the West Coast of the South Island. Stepping outside our motel, my wife Jenny, my support worker Leuila Letoga and I were blessed with a spectacular vista of Franz Josef Glacier (Kā Roimata o Hine Hukatere) rising high into the Great Divide (picture 11).

We were about to make an ascent by helicopter over the backbone of New Zealand, including the highest mountain peaks which separate the East Coast from the West Coast, one of the last of our adventures on a South Island holiday in the summer of 2019-2020. We had achieved everything I had planned up until this point, and my heart was buzzing with hope for the event that was about to unfold. A wet weather front was rolling in the next day, and we were only staying in Franz Josef for three nights. If we couldn't fly that day, the opportunity might not present itself again. The sky was clear, filling me with gratitude and excitement about the flight.

I'd been up in a helicopter several times before as a youth in the 1980s. The first trip was a brief pleasure flight from Waihi Beach while on holiday with Mum and Dad, and the second was with my mate Grant Sims at the National Fieldays at Mystery Creek near Hamilton. I won this as a spot prize in one of their competitions. My third flight was the first in my current condition when I shared a short 15-minute flight over Rotorua Lakes with former company HeliPro. In each case I thoroughly enjoyed the sensation of flight and contrast to a fixed wing aircraft.

We had booked our adventure through Makingtrax and Helicopter Line which flies out of Franz Josef Village and other South Island locations. Makingtrax was set up by adventure junkie Jezza Williams. In 2010, the same year of my accident, Jezza was working as a canyoning instructor in Switzerland when he slipped on a rock and fell, sustaining a high-level spinal injury similar to mine. Just a couple of years later, he set up a business to facilitate adventure opportunities for people with disabilities to enjoy. Pretty impressive! He is one of the only certified quadriplegic hang gliders in the world, not letting physical limitations override his ability to enjoy life. He says, "I just wanna keep on rockin'."[2]

The night before, we had asked my support worker Leuila if she was up for a surprise, to which she responded, "Yes!" Leuila is a lovely Samoan lady who has been the longest serving member of my support team. She started in 2012, after covering a shift for someone else, and has remained ever since. She drives over from Tokoroa to Rotorua each week for several shifts. This helicopter flight was an adventure for her as well. She had never been up in a helicopter or in snow before, so Jenny and I were glad to share the experience with her, and she became the envy of all her family and friends when they found out later what she'd done. She had gone to bed the night before, wondering if we were going bungee jumping! I'm up for a challenge, but I'm not sure my body would sustain that degree of stress!

So, that morning, after checking in at the Helicopter Line base and investigating the route, we headed off down to the helicopter pad with Brendan, a cheerful West Coaster who accompanied us on the flight and assisted with my needs. Helicopter Line made an exception to book the whole helicopter just for us. Brendan took the seat normally assigned to another paying customer. Jenny sat in the front seat to the left of the pilot, with Brendan and Leuila in the back next to me.

While the propeller blades idled gently, I positioned my wheelchair alongside the helicopter. It wasn't pretty, but Brendan picked me up out of the wheelchair and placed me in the rear seat of the helicopter (picture 12). He was as strong as an ox, with legs like tree trunks, and the only person to have ever carried a dead weight like me on his own without any assistance from a hoist! I don't weigh myself very often, thank goodness! At best guess, I would have been around 90 to 95 kilograms, which Brendan tackled capably.

Off we went, soaring steadily upward and alongside the 12-kilometre-long Franz Josef Glacier, which has the lowest terminal face elevation of any glacier flowing into a rainforest in the world. The flight was calmer than I'd expected, the gentle alpine breeze barely noticeable inside the AS355 Squirrel helicopter. I felt relieved that we were finally on our way. We landed on top of the glacier as planned, approximately 2,500 metres (8,200 feet) above sea level.

Brendan unfolded a sled which had been mounted on the helicopter skids for me. Essentially, this was my skis, specially designed by Jezza. Brendan lifted me out of the helicopter and onto the small seat which had been mounted onto the skis. Having dressed for the Alpine environment, I was pleasantly surprised at how warm and still the air was. This was the first time I'd been on snow since before my accident in 2010 (picture 13). It was an emotional moment, the culmination of many phone calls and thorough planning in the months before.

I desperately missed the snow. I was by no means an expert skier but had skied most winters since young adulthood, usually on Mount Ruapehu in the Tongariro National Park, but also during a brief trip with my mates in the late 1980s when we tackled some of the South Island fields: Mount Hutt, The Remarkables, Cardrona, and Treble Cone. This time I was seated on three skis instead of standing on two! It didn't matter to me; I was on the snow.

It was heaps of fun on the glacier. Brendan and the pilot didn't rush us but pushed me around on the snow until they ran out of puff. My disability didn't seem a barrier to being able to enjoy the environment. I can relate to comments made by Jezza:

> I'm quite disabled, if you like. And that means, if I can do it, then anybody can do it. If it's not possible, I'll make it possible. And, if somebody says no. Then, I will defy what they think. And I'll make sure that they go: oh, oh, okay, this is possible.[3]

This was the highest I had ever skied on a New Zealand slope. I'm not going to apologise for stretching the metaphor; it was still skiing! My previous dream of heliskiing one day in the Harris Mountains near Wānaka was now a distant memory. Sad that may be, but I was making a new memory from which to share in the days and months ahead.

We had decided to pay for the longer flight around the top of Mount Cook, down over Fox Glacier before returning to Franz Josef. However, we had been warned that this wasn't guaranteed, given the fragility of the alpine conditions at altitude. Furthermore, the pilot told us they had only been able to fly 40 percent of the summer so far due to poor weather conditions.

When we got back in the helicopter (thanks to another lift from Brendan), the pilot assessed the weather conditions and told us that it was safe enough to continue with the longer flight – Yippee! So we took off from the glacier, flying up and over the Great Divide. Our altitude enabled us to see a snippet of the East Coast on the horizon and the West Coast behind us at the same time.

To gain further elevation, the pilot circled out over Tasman Glacier, up and around to the northern side of Aoraki Mount Cook which, at 3,724 metres (12,218 feet), is New Zealand's highest peak. One of the tramping huts we could see below us appeared like a matchbox halfway down the mountain. As we continued our way around the summit, we felt we could reach out and touch it. We were literally at the top of New Zealand and, as the pilot informed us, flying close to the limits of our Squirrel helicopter. I would remember these moments with awe and gratitude for a long time.

Within five minutes or so, we had almost circumnavigated Mount Cook, though it seemed slower at altitude, almost as if we were standing still, and the world was rotating around us. We began our descent southwest until Fox Glacier (town) came into view. Then we progressed slowly back around the lower reaches of the beach forest and returned to the helicopter base beside the Waiho River. The flight had taken about 50 minutes in total.

After one more lift for Brendan, I was back into my wheels on the ground. Both he and the pilot had taken wonderful care of us throughout the whole trip. I was conscious of how expensive it is to run a helicopter, yet their body language was reassuringly relaxed. Our pilot told us he was in the job because he wanted to facilitate adventures for people just like me. The Kiwi 'can do' attitude is alive and well!

That afternoon, we drove around the winding roads to nearby Lake Matheson, hoping to see its famous, often-photographed mountain reflections. It's only about 30 minutes' walk from the car park through pretty, native New Zealand bush, easily manageable in my wheelchair (picture 14). By now, the afternoon cloud was rolling in, so it wasn't quite the vista we were hoping for. Nonetheless, still buzzing from the earlier flight, we enjoyed the flora and fauna of the West Coast bush.

What an awesome day – it filled us with joy and gratitude! God had blessed us with wonderful weather and the opportunity to visit the highest reaches of New Zealand within a very short window of time. It was the flight of a lifetime, filling me with so much hope and reminding me that many things were still possible despite my disability. I felt there were no limits to what I could achieve if I put my mind to it. Even today, if somebody tells me something can't be done, I generally don't accept that. As the saying goes, "Where there's a will, there's a way."

I'm reminded of a visit to a parishioner in the early days

after my accident. He had a split-level home and was determined that I could make it upstairs. I had to wheel across the rose garden, up my two-metre-long ramps, over some concrete steps, through the front door and into the entranceway. Then, I straddled two-metre-long laminated painting beams with each of my driving wheels, up the stairway into the lounge and dining room! Imagine the paperwork if I fell!

People who think inclusively are like gold, and I'm grateful to my host that day, Neil Gumbley, for his Kiwi ingenuity. I was, and continue to be determined not to dig a hole and hide away behind closed doors in a state of depression. There is always hope, no matter what my situation. The opportunities are endless; especially when people like Jezza exist, helping people like me explore and enjoy all the natural beauty that New Zealand has to offer.

Another adventure story involves a group of dads like myself, all united in having a child with neurodiverse needs: autism, attention deficit hyperactivity disorder, Tourette syndrome, and the like. Funding organised by Parent to Parent enabled us to share an outdoor experience together, run by Off Road NZ, situated on a rural property near Mamaku. On Saturday 9 November 2024, Jenny, Hamish, Callum and I set out from Rotorua to meet the other guys.

We were booked on the 'Monster 4×4 Thrill Ride'. The specially adapted Jeep was set high above the ground, powered by a 3.8-litre Holden Commodore engine. It had four-wheel steering and large chunky tyres for improved traction.

To get me on board, the guys had to use my sling to lift me out of my electric wheelchair, off the raised deck, under the rollbar and into the centre seat where I was secured by full harness restraints. I'm completely vulnerable in situations like this, having learnt to relax in the moment and trust those looking out for my comfort and safety. It took some manoeuvring to bend my legs sufficiently to clear the side of the vehicle while sliding my back over the edges of the seat. I had bought my special cushion to give my skin some protection on the hard plastic racing seats.

Once I was in, the boys sat either side of me and gripped my sling to stop me sliding around. Normally, without the necessary nerve function to use the muscles in my hands effectively, my fingers would slip off the front bar. But the boys held my hands in place, giving me some stability. It felt so precious to be enjoying this experience with my two sons.

We set off, and I was immediately conscious that this was going to be a rough ride. It had been some time since I'd given my body such a rigorous shake across a gravel track in a rural bush setting. We moved somewhat more quickly than I had imagined, at least until the first obstacle. It reminded me of riding motorbikes and tractors in my earlier years on the farm, something we wouldn't have thought twice about then. We made our way through steep gullies, over wooden barriers, and down specially designed contoured obstacles which included a 70-degree incline.

We went down first, then made our way back up the same steep incline. It had steel ramps with serrated edges set into the bank so the tyres could maintain enough traction for us to navigate the obstacle successfully. It felt like we were almost vertical, and the vehicle was going to roll at any moment. The back tyres slipped for a few seconds just before we made our way back onto the bush track. We were completely reliant on the skill of the driver and our highly specialised vehicle. What a relief to enter the next part of the track!

We were back soon enough, smiles all round. The boys noticed that one of my shoes had partially fallen off and exposed my heel to a metal bar on the floor of the vehicle. Hamish was worried about the mark on my skin. Fortunately, it had gone away by the next morning, though I had a few small bruises, one on my foot and the other on my left shoulder. It didn't matter to me, even if my skin took some time to recover. I was pushing the boundaries of what my body could tolerate, yet again!

Hamish said to me later that I must've been pumping enough adrenaline to achieve what would normally be a near impossible feat in my condition.

As we got back into the van, we all talked excitedly about the experience and which parts were the most thrilling. At that moment my emotions got the better of me. I was so blessed to have experienced this adventure with both boys by my side.

My family has been a wonderful mainstay for me. Hamish often drops tools and comes to my aid – literally, because he is a builder! After renovating our upstairs bathroom over the summer of 2016, I offered to gift him a shared parasailing adventure with Kawerau Jet to say thank you.

This took some planning as the weather had to be calm enough for the boat to skim smoothly across the lake with sufficient speed to catch the wind in our chute above. On Sunday 13 March 2016 we ventured down to the lake. Friends gathered on the shore to watch. One of the staff even grabbed the other jet boat and took several of them out to film the experience at no extra cost. No doubt it was a novel experience for them to entertain a crazy bloke with a spinal injury who was still willing to take a risk and give something a go.

My level of injury was the highest of any client they had taken out before! It was too scary for Jenny. She couldn't cope with the idea of me dangling precariously 50 metres above the water. She was also unsure how I would get back on the boat without damaging my legs. So she stayed at home and watched it all on video later.

The staff came up with an ingenious way to seat me comfortably in the back of the boat. The boss leapt into the shallow water beside the wharf and fished out an old plastic chair. He proceeded to chop the legs off with a skill saw, then sat it inside the safety rails of the boat for me to perch on. That provided some amusement for those watching!

Friends and family secured my life jacket and wrapped me in my sling, at which point they manhandled me into the boat and down onto the plastic chair. My brother Steve and friend Ian Jackson kept me stable until the time came for our ascent. A staff member on the boat harnessed me to Hamish in preparation for the flight. It was quite scary exiting the rear of the boat, flopping forward in my harness and lurching out over the water. Hamish reassured me by saying, "I've got you Dad."

We were blessed with a brilliant panorama over the city and surrounding hills (picture 15). At the end of the 'flight', the pilot usually slows down to drop the parasailers as close to the water as possible without them falling in. In our case, Steve was freaking out in the boat, telling them to speed up and not attempt to put us anywhere near the water. I thought we were fine, and felt confident to be living on the edge in that moment.

Then the time came to bring us back into the boat. Bear in mind that I have limited movement in my legs. Just as we were coming in to land, one of my legs momentarily caught the back edge of the boat. I was grateful that Steve and Ian were there to lift us safely onto the platform. Our friends in the other jet boat cheered as the pilot slowed the winch and lowered us down safely. We'd made it back safely without drowning or breaking any bones!

A week later Jenny and I took a cake to say thank you to the Kawarau Jet staff, which they appreciated. A month later, I spoke to Fiona who owned and ran the business with her husband Ross for 12 years. He often skippered the launch boat. Fiona informed me that on an outing only a few weeks after our adventure, the main rope to the parachute had broken! This had never happened for them before, although it has occurred a couple of times since.

For me, it was another experience that wouldn't have happened without the support of family and friends. Jenny knows there are other adventure activities I've yet to tick off my bucket list! One of them is tandem paragliding, having watched people doing this from the top of Treble Cone ski field near Wānaka. I have reached out to a local proprietor to see if it can happen here in the Bay of Plenty from the top of Mount Maunganui. Watch this space!

I continue to enjoy life, perhaps pushing the boundaries for someone with my level of injury yet still determined to give things a go if I can see a way of making it happen. There is so much scope for enjoying the outdoors in New Zealand, despite one's physical or mental vulnerabilities. I'm living proof of that, operating each day by the grace of God and holding to absolute hope and promise in Him.

Questions for reflection:

What activity or experience would you consider doing despite your physical or mental limitations? How might you gain the courage to bring that to fulfilment?

If money was no object, what activity would you participate in, and how might you involve others in celebrating that experience with you?

How has New Zealand's natural environment contributed to and enriched your journey?

Chapter 10

Maybe Tomorrow Isn't So Bad After All!

According to Snyder's Hope Theory, hope is supported by having a realistic goal, multiple pathways to reach it, and a sense of agency, that is, a belief that I can follow the pathways.
– Lucy Hone[1]

If I'm honest, my goals are very fluid because I'm involved with a variety of different community groups, seasonal focuses, supervision expectations, speaking engagements, recreational activities, and so on. I like being flexible, as it fits with my lifestyle.

For example, our Sailability group hosted a national regatta in February 2024. I looked forward to it and was grateful to our members for making it happen. My friend Phil skippered our dinghy, as he's done many times over the years. He is an experienced sailor and inspires confidence when we are out on the water. It was the first time we'd competed, jostling for the start line with other competitors and reading the wind patterns, just as you see the tactician doing for Team New Zealand on the bigger boats.

This event benefited others with disabilities like mine and it was fulfilling for me to participate in a gathering centred around a sport that is such a passion for many New Zealanders. When the regatta was over, we gathered at the foreshore to share stories, enjoy barbecue food, and give prizes to the best teams. I took delight in encouraging the participants and hosting with our local volunteers, who willingly gave time and energy to make it all happen.

In each of my different focus groups, I've made valuable connections with other Kiwis which have opened up mutual pathways of hope and encouragement. I would not have envisioned this happening in the early stages after my accident. Then, I was still numb as I grappled with my new reality, unsure how the future would unfold and questioning my place alongside others in wheelchairs.

I'm comfortable now in this new venture, happy to keep exploring new pathways of significance as they arise, but I recognise the value of the road travelled so far – the heritage of my early years, plus the fruitful and difficult seasons which have helped to shape my identity as a proud Kiwi.

My support team, whom I greatly appreciate, are loyal to my needs and a valuable support in our household. I would not be able to do everything I do if I was just reliant on Jenny, our family and friends. My support workers are mostly immigrants, from a rich diversity of cultural backgrounds. I have sought to learn snippets of their languages, to both honour their culture and bolster my own.

My longest-standing support worker, Leuila Letoga, taught me a proverb from her Samoan culture some years ago. It goes like this: "O le tagata ma lona fa'asinomaga," meaning, "Everyone has a heritage, and place of identity."

I've endeavoured to be honest about who I am, my family background, my faith, my achievements and my weaknesses. I'm shaped by the past, and secure in my future. Furthermore,

I've sought to highlight that our vulnerabilities and struggles need not be endpoints or result in never-ending bad days; instead, they are realities that we can embrace and use to build hopeful resilience.

> Hope invites us to recognize the reality, the suffering and struggle in this life, but at the very same time to know deeply that our suffering and our struggles do not have the last word. (Henri Nouwen)[2]

I love the power of a good story, and the different genres used to tell it, particularly a movie that unpacks real-life struggles. While on holiday at Ōhope Beach recently, Jenny and I watched a movie called *Tinā* at nearby Whakatane. The story is filmed in Christchurch and inspired by true events; the main character, Mareta, is a Samoan teacher, a godmother to the people of her community and an advocate for Pasifika education, her heritage and place of identity.

Mareta is grief-stricken by the loss of her daughter in the February 2011 Christchurch earthquake and as her mental health declines, she becomes unemployed. Eventually she is forced to apply for a job and secures a position at an elite private school. Despite being a 'fish out of water' socially and culturally, Mareta discovers many of her students are also traumatised by the earthquake and other life experiences, especially a young woman called Sophie who becomes almost a substitute daughter.

Against opposition from the school's conservative, sports-focused hierarchy, Mareta starts a choir and encourages her students to participate in the upcoming Big Sing school choir competition. Through her coaching, and inspired by her culture, the choir members discover the value of community and support for each other. At the same time, Mareta rediscovers her passion for teaching and mothering others.

The movie is a tearjerker, as I discovered. It ends – spoiler alert! – with Mareta dying, but Sophie finding new confidence and self-worth in leading the choir at the Big Sing, in spite of her physical and emotional scars.

By the end of the movie, tears were streaming down my face and Jenny had to wipe them from my cheeks. I found myself being drawn into Mareta and Sophie's shared grief, a reflection of the deep relationship they had built. In those moments, I knew that some of my tears reflected my own grief and loss.

> *The wounds feel less tender in time, but they are still wounds. The memories fade after a while, the reminders can bring them back in a moment.*[3]

But I was also inspired, watching the faces of the choir members – hope-filled and encouraged, singing with all the emotion and passion they could muster. This is what drives me – community and togetherness, investing in others, instilling hope and seeing the difference it makes for them, despite my own grief and suffering.

Hope means being real about our present suffering but anticipating that seasons do change, and new horizons emerge. Coming to terms with our suffering can be foundational to building new ventures which may be beneficial to others on their own journeys. We can help construct pathways of hope for those to whom we seek to minister and serve. However, our journey thus far should never be forgotten – the nurturing and learning, the tangible and intangible, the spiritual and the cultural aspects. That's why I appreciate Leuila's Samoan proverb: "Everyone has a heritage, and place of identity."

My life before tetraplegia is of vital importance to me – the things I've learnt, my heritage, my family and those involved in shaping it. The values I hold dear have been established in the past yet honed more profoundly through enduring the most difficult life circumstances.

If I focus on the glaringly obvious ugly stuff that impacts me today, I can risk losing sight of progress made. I can forget to acknowledge those who have given me hope during the toughest times. Yes, I am left with scars that trigger difficult memories, regrets and ongoing frustrations. They are real! Yet the journey so far has enabled me to paint (metaphorically) a rich piece of landscape art. This landscape is only made possible through acknowledging my memory of 'before' and what has unfolded 'after' my accident – aspects of my experience that will always be in tension, but which enable me to understand others who travel a similar road.

In other words, our unique perspective gives depth to the road travelled by others.

Seeing one's suffering in perspective is essential for cultivating self-awareness, gratitude, empathy, and growth outside of our tendency towards self-focus.[4]

Author and 24-7 prayer leader Pete Greig tells the story of art critic Robert Cumming's experience when viewing a painting by 16th century Renaissance master Filippino Lippi in the National Gallery of London. It depicts Mary the mother of Jesus with baby Jesus on her lap and two saints, Jerome and Dominic, kneeling at her feet. *The Virgin and Child with Saints*

Jerome and Dominic (c.1485) has never been regarded as Lippi's best work, because the perspective gives the impression that the mountains behind Mary are about to topple over. However, as Cumming discovered, a fresh perspective drew him deeper into Lippi's intentions for his work.

> Robert Cumming was standing analysing this painting one day ... and he had an epiphany. He suddenly realised it wasn't painted to hang in an art gallery. ...it was painted as an altarpiece. So, very self-consciously the proud art critic knelt down on the marble floor in front of this second-rate painting, very aware of everyone around him. But he said, as he did so, the whole painting morphed and came into perfect perspective. And he found himself kneeling between St Jerome and St Dominic looking up at Christ, up at Mary, up at this scene. And everything came into perfect perspective.[5]

My uncle's painting, mentioned earlier, is a landscape full of beauty, reminding me of a period in history that is full of great memories. It also makes me incredibly grateful for the opportunities I had when fully fit and able-bodied, training as an athlete and sharing that rural environment with extended family, friends and neighbours. Therefore, the difficult things of tomorrow don't seem so bad when seen from the perspective of the many blessings I experienced in the place I came from.

Yet, I also remain grounded in my present reality, enough to care for myself, and be a help to others on similar journeys in our community. At the same time, I'm keeping one eye on the future as an avenue of hope beyond this broken world of ours. That's an enduring perspective I trust will help you survive your present reality too. As C.S. Lewis wrote:

Hope is one of the theological virtues. This means that a continual looking forward to the eternal world is not (as some modern people think) a form of escapism or wishful thinking, but one of the things that a Christian is meant to do. It does not mean that we are to leave the present world as it is. If you read history, you will find that the Christians who did most for the present world were just those who thought most of the next.[6]

There is always so much more to be done, and so much despair when considering what we could change or do differently if we had the time over again. But that kind of thinking is also a form of escapism because it denies the opportunity to be grateful for what we've achieved, and to build resilience and tenacity through the difficult times in our lives. That's a daily choice for me despite my struggles. I like what psychologist Brené Brown has to say in this regard:

In my work, I found that moving out of powerlessness, and even despair, requires hope. Hope is not an emotion: it's a cognitive process – a thought process made up of what researcher C.R. Snyder called the trilogy of "goals, pathways, and agency." Hope happens when we can set goals, have the tenacity and perseverance to pursue those goals, and believe in our own abilities to act. Snyder also found that hope is learned. When boundaries, consistency, and support are in place, children learn it from their parents. But even if we didn't get it as kids, we can still learn hope as adults. It's just tougher when we are older because we have to resist and unlearn old habits, like the tendency to give up when things get tough. Hope is a function of struggle. If we are never allowed to fail or face adversity as children, we are denied the opportunity to develop the tenacity

> and sense of agency we need to be hopeful. One of the greatest gifts my parents gave me was hope.[7]

My goal in penning these words has been to impart hope to you, the reader; to lift your sights beyond the tough things you've endured, and to show that it is possible to forge new pathways of significance, despite experiencing traumatic and challenging events. A new pathway doesn't mean losing your unique identity and calling. It will however, as I have discovered, deepen your understanding of God's plan for your life and give you fresh resolve to travel the journey with others, whatever their horizon.

> Our suffering is bigger than ourselves, but our healing is bigger than ourselves too. This is why community is absolutely necessary in the redefining of our calling. We'll never know the biggest vision God has for our lives in this world until we see that vision reflected in someone else's story. We'll never gain a true perspective on all we've been given and all we'll never be able to do by ourselves, until we open our deepest hopes and fears to each other.[8]

Every day of every week of every year carries hope if we consider the small things, like waking to the sound of tūī in the trees or taking the opportunity to smile or be smiled at – in my case, especially by my adorable grandson!

Some people don't have the things that many of us take for granted, like food on the table, a roof over our head and good mental health. Others whom I encounter regularly in our community, can't escape cycles of abuse, poverty or violence. Hope is realised for them if I pay attention, help with their basic needs and lift their spirits by conveying warm messages of encouragement and care. In my limited capacity, I feel that I can only do a little towards meeting fellow humans' needs, but I must at least try to make a difference for their survival when opportunity presents itself.

I like the analogy of the old man walking along the shoreline after a storm. He discovered a vast number of starfish lying washed up on the beach in every direction. He noticed a small boy walking towards him, pausing occasionally to pick up a starfish and throw it into the sea. The old man commented to the boy, "Surely your efforts won't make much difference, because many will die when the sun takes effect." The boy bent down, picked up another starfish and threw it into the ocean. "There you are," he said, "it made a difference to that one!"

In the 2018 movie *Ready Player One*, one of the characters called Halliday wants to escape reality through a simulation game. There is an oasis in the game where players can go to avoid battles. Halliday's friend Wade wants to stay at the oasis to avoid the consequences of warfare and conflict. However, when he witnesses the suffering of his friend Samantha back in the real world, and acknowledges how much he cares for her, he realises that he should leave his quiet place and fight alongside her on the battlefield.

We can't solve the problems of all those around us who struggle to find an oasis from life's battles. But we can make a difference for one at a time. We can journey with them, seek to understand their needs, fight for them, and alleviate their suffering as much as we are able. We can give them respite and show compassion in the fragility of life. By doing so, we begin to understand each other better and therefore adopt a shared sense of suffering which gives way to a hopeful horizon.

> *Our human compassion binds us the one to the other, not in pity or patronising, but as human beings who have learnt how to turn our common suffering into hope for the future.* (Nelson Mandela)[9]

I worship the God who resurrected life itself through the actions of His Son Jesus Christ on the cross. That gives me hope and shows me there is a larger dimension to the cosmos than I can comprehend. Nonetheless, I'm determined to walk the journey of faith, trusting as best as I can in my heavenly Father who knows, sees, hears and loves. He's proven to be faithful, gracious and loving to me when I fall short.

When I wake up each morning to the complex issues, difficult realities and challenges of our lives in this 21st century, I can only conclude that there has to be something outside what I see with my physical eyes – a hope that takes me beyond what I struggle to understand. I guess that's why the apostle Paul sought to open the minds of those he lived with and fill them with something of that larger dimension.

> *So, we fix our eyes not on what is seen, but on what is unseen, since what is seen is temporary, and what is unseen is eternal.* (2 Corinthians 4:18)

You and I are both on a journey with God whether we believe it or not. We share this cosmos together, carry the same capacity to love or hate, to frame our tomorrows with darkness or light, to make the effort to get up in the morning and fight for our fellow human beings instead of creating destruction for them. There is always a choice in how we respond to what's happening in the cosmos, whether it affects us personally or our neighbours in local communities and beyond.

Can I humbly suggest that a loving and generous approach to life will help us to stay in this battle? It's no easier to say than it is to practise, if I'm honest. But the Christian faith gives me the strength to have a go and paints a picture of pathways of hope toward the horizon. Would you join me on that journey, entertain a future filled with new and fulfilling possibilities, gain a fresh perspective alongside others, perhaps choose a different pathway for your own life? It's not easy, but it's worth it!

Live a life filled with love, following the example of Christ. He loved and offered Himself as a sacrifice for us, a pleasing aroma to God. (Ephesians 5:2, NLT)

Questions for reflection:

What gets you up in the morning? How could you be a channel of love, hope and generosity in your world?

Who could you reach out to who would help you explore the Christian faith?

Is there one person for whom you could make a difference? Think about one person to whom you could 'pay it forward' and breathe hope into their life.

Notes

Preface

1. New Zealand Spinal Cord Injury Registry. From: nzspinaltrust. org.nz/i-need-information/new-zealand-spinal-cord-injury-registry-nzscir/nzscir-statistics/ Acknowledgements: The authors thank the New Zealand Spinal Cord Injury Registry and both Auckland and Christchurch sites. NZSCIR is modelled on the Canadian Rick Hansen Spinal Cord Injury Registry (RHSCIR) in collaboration with the Praxis Spinal Cord Institute.
2. Health and Well-Being statistics. (2021). World Health Organisation. From: www.who.int/data/gho/data/major-themes/health-and-well-being

Chapter 1: Rich Beginnings and the Call of God

1. Holtey, T. 'The Importance of Storytelling for a Hospice Chaplain.' Hospice Red River Valley. www.hrrv.org/blog/the-importance-of-storytelling-for-a-hospice-chaplain/
2. Luther, M. cited in Crocker, M. (23 November). 'What Authority Does a Government Have? Let's ask Luther.' Christ City Network. christcitychurch.ca/media/what-authority-does-a-government-have-lets-ask-luther/

Chapter 2: When Life Changes in a Flash

1. Nouwen, H. (1996). *The Inner Voice of Love: A Journey through Anguish to Freedom*. Bantam Doubleday. (p. 38)

2. Casting Crowns. (2005). 'Praise You in This Storm' (song). *Lifesong* (album), Beach Street Records and Reunion Records.
3. Koziol, C. (2021). 'Journaling's Impact on Mental Health.' *UWL Journal of Undergraduate Research*, 24. (p. 2) www.uwlax.edu/globalassets/offices-services/urc/jur-online/pdf/2021/koziol.callie.eng.pdf Koziol also refers to a study conducted by Phillips, Lynne and Rolfe (2016), which finds that the discipline of writing is a means of catharsis. They also note that writing enables self-expression, which may not be immediately accessible when first explored.
4. Watson, E. quoted in *Jimazing Thoughts*. (September 8, 2013) 'Living Presence'. jimazing.com/2013/09/08/living-presence/
5. I Am They. (2018). 'Scars'(song). *Trial and Triumph* (album), Essential Records.
6. Ember, A. 'Grief and loss.' Healthify. Reviewed 13 September 2022. healthify.nz/health-a-z/g/grief-loss/#:~:text=Grief%20is%20the%20natural%20reaction,loved%20one%20or%20your%20employment.
7. Nouwen, H. (8 July, 2006). *Bread for the Journey: A Daybook of Wisdom and Faith*. HarperSanFrancisco.

Chapter 3: People Really Do Care

1. Hone, L. (2016). *What Abi Taught Us: A mother's struggle to come to terms with her daughter's death*. Allen & Unwin. (p. 121)
2. Yancey, P. (1990). *Where is God when it Hurts?* Zondervan. (pp. 176-177)
3. Tedeschi, R. cited in Hone, (2016). (p. 213)
4. Noel, J. (2015). *Message to My Girl*. Allen & Unwin. (p. 205)
5. Nouwen, H. (2004). *Out of Solitude: Three Meditations on the Christian Life*. Ave Maria Press. (p. 34)
6. Waldinger, R., & Schulz, M. (2023). *The Good Life and How to Live It*. Ebury. (p. 116).

7. Gass, B. (3 September 2016). *Word for Today*. Rhema Media.
8. 'What Matters to You?' (2018-2025). Department of Health, Western Australia. smhs.health.wa.gov.au/Our-care/Safe-quality-care/What-matters-to-you
9. Wolf, J., & Wolf, K. (2020). *Suffer Strong: How to Survive Anything by Redefining Everything*. HarperCollins. (p. 23)
10. 'Te Whare Tapa Whā.' Mental Health Foundation of New Zealand. mentalhealth.org.nz/te-whare-tapa-wha
11. 'Five Ways to Wellbeing.' Mental Health Foundation of New Zealand. mentalhealth.org.nz/five-ways-to-wellbeing
12. 'All Right?' Mental Health Foundation of New Zealand and Canterbury District Health Board. www.allright.org.nz/ Note: The app is no longer available.
13. Boren, Cindy. (18 August 2016) 'Abbey D'Agostino and Nikki Hamblin 'Olympic spirit' moment: Reality hits with runner's knee injury.' *Sydney Morning Herald*. www.smh.com.au/sport/abbey-dagostino-and-nikki-hamblin-olympic-spirit-moment-reality-hits-with-runners-knee-injury-20160818-gqv3i7.html
14. Williams, D. (16 August 2017). 'Catch up with Inspiring Olympians Nikki Hamblin Abbey D'Agostino.' ESPN. www.espn.com/olympics/story/_/id/20278032/catch-inspiring-olympians-nikki-hamblin-abbey-dagostino-one-year-collision-rio
15. Mother Teresa. (1997). *The Joy in Loving: A guide to everyday living*. Compiled by Jaya Chalika and Edward Le Joly. Penguin Books.

Chapter 4: Getting the Right Help

1. Lowry, A. (20 April 2022). 'Amanda Lowry Keynote.' New Zealand Health Group. YouTube. (8:45-9:00). www.youtube.com/watch?v=q0La_ErdwRU
2. 'Annual report: ACC supports 2 million new claims in 50th year.' (16 Oct 2024) ACC Newsroom. www.acc.co.nz/newsroom/stories/annual-report-acc-supports-2-million-new-claims-in-50th-year

3. 'Five Ways to Wellbeing: A best practice guide.' Mental Health Foundation of New Zealand. mentalhealth.org.nz/resources/resource/five-ways-to-wellbeing-best-practice-guide

4. ibid.

5. Wilson, M. (23 July 2022). 'Tauranga paraplegic left without care due to 'severe' support worker shortage.' *Bay of Plenty Times*.

6. ibid.

7. Lowry, A. (20 April 2022). 'Amanda Lowry Keynote.' New Zealand Health Group. *YouTube*. (13:24-13:26). www.youtube.com/watch?v=q0La_ErdwRU

8. Wilson, M. (23 July 2022). 'Tauranga paraplegic left without care due to 'severe' support worker shortage.' *Bay of Plenty Times*.

9. Beutler, T.M., & Chin, L. (2024). 'Spinal Cord Injuries.' Medscape. emedicine.medscape.com/article/793582-overview#a6?form=fpf Note: Requires a login to access.

10. McDonald, R. (8 January 2015). 'Family Carers Case – Five Years On.' Public Address: Access disability and different worlds. publicaddress.net/access/family-carers-case-five-years-on/

11. Cited in ibid.

12. 'Fact sheet: For people receiving Disability Support Services. Version 1.4' (23 September 2024). Whaikaha Ministry of Disabled People. www.whaikaha.govt.nz/news/independent-review/fact-sheet-for-people-receiving-dss

13. Doocey, Hon M. (12 December 2024). 'Independent Review of ACC Announced.' Beehive.govt.nz Releases. www.beehive.govt.nz/release/independent-review-acc-announced

14. Stephen Hawking Quotes. (n.d.). BrainyQuote.com. www.brainyquote.com/quotes/stephen_hawking_627103 (Accessed 28 August 2024).

Chapter 5: Finding My Place in an Unfamiliar World

1. Fosslien, L., & Duffy, M.W. (2019). *No Hard Feelings: The secret power of embracing emotions at work*. Penguin. (p. 185)

2. Singer, Bryan (Dir). (2016). *X-Men Apocalypse* (Film). 20th Century Studios.

3. Lowry, A. (20 April 2022). 'Amanda Lowry Keynote.' New Zealand Health Group. *YouTube*. (11:02-11:11). www.youtube.com/watch?v=qoLa_ErdwRU

4. Myers, J. (2003). *The Search to Belong: Rethinking Intimacy, Community and Small Groups*. Zondervan. (p. 26)

5. 'Whakatauki Information Sheet.' (2019). Inspiring Communities. inspiringcommunities.org.nz/wp-content/uploads/2019/03/Inspiring-Communities-%E2%80%93-Whakatauki-information-sheet.pdf. (p. 1)

6. Lowry, A. (20 April 2022). 'Amanda Lowry Keynote.' New Zealand Health Group. *YouTube*. (3:12-3:15). www.youtube.com/watch?v=qoLa_ErdwRU

7. Suicide data web tool. Health New Zealand Te Whatu Ora. tewhatuora.shinyapps.io/suicide-web-tool/

8. 'Housing Modification (HMOD) and Housing Assessment (HMA) Services: Operational Guidelines.' (March 2025). ACC. www.acc.co.nz/assets/provider/Housing-Modification-and-Housing-Assessment-Services-Operational-Guidelines.pdf

9. Garcia, M. (25 July 2022). 'Whaikaha: The new Ministry of Disabled people inspires hopes for empowerment.' *Rotorua Daily Post*. www.nzherald.co.nz/rotorua-daily-post/news/whaikaha-the-new-ministry-of-disabled-people-inspires-hopes-for-empowerment/SGWHPGPIVI3FVHOK2FZZVNMGMA/

10. 'Welcome.' (n.d.) Elevate Christian Disability Trust. elevatecdt.org.nz

11. 'Appendix: disabled people population and life outcome statistics.' 2024 *Pūrongo ā-tau Annual Report*. Whaikaha Ministry of Disabled People. www.whaikaha.govt.nz/about-us/corporate-publications/annual-reports/annual-report-2024/appendix

12. Habets, M. (2016). 'Disability and Divinization: Eschatological Parables and Allegations.' In A. Picard & M. Habets (Eds). *Theology and the Experience of Disability Interdisciplinary: Perspectives from Voices Down Under*. Routledge. (pp. 212-234)

13. Murray Sheard Podcast. (6 November 2023). 'Charles Hewlett: Holding discomfort.' Faith, Church & Disability. CBM. Available on Spotify: open.spotify.com/episode/0qCeGOFgoZWQxdXTWbIOzR?si=HyhD75jUToSp68puDUegIQ

14. Barratt, I. (15 February 2017). 'More than able.' *War Cry* magazine, 11 February 2017 (pp. 6-9). www.salvationarmy.org.nz/more-than-able/

15. Quoted in 'Pride of NZ awards local heroes – who's your inspiration' (1 September 2015). *New Zealand Herald*. www.nzherald.co.nz/nz/pride-of-nz-awards-local-heroes-whos-your-inspiration/J6XWW3CUKIOHPEGU5CEL53KZEY/

16. 'Whakatauki Information Sheet.' (2019). (p. 5)

17. ibid.

Chapter 6: Where is God When Bad Things Happen?

1. Przybys, J. (9 April 2010). '"Shack" author surprised by success.' *Las Vegas Review-Journal*. www.reviewjournal.com/news/shack-author-surprised-by-success/

2. Wortman, C., cited in Hone, L. (2016). (p. 100)

3. Kluger, J. (31 July 2012). 'A Breakthrough at Last for Spinal-Cord-Injury Research?' *Time Magazine*. healthland.time.com/2012/07/31/a-breakthrough-at-last-for-spinal-cord-injury-research/

4. Lewis, C.S. (2001). *The Problem of Pain*. HarperOne. (p. 22)

5. Frankl, V.E. (2014). *Man's Search for Meaning*. (original Ger., 1946, original Eng. trans, 1959; Boston Press, 2014). (p. 62)

6. 'Episode 1: Tony Quinn' (17 November 2020) Origin Stories with Robert Tighe. *YouTube* (29:09-29:12). www.youtube.com/watch?v=XpsKBPNZmmo

7. Allport, G. (1964). Preface. In Frankl, V.E. (2014). (p. 9)

8. 'Maya Angelou quotes: 15 of the best.' (29 May 2014) *The Guardian*. www.theguardian.com/books/2014/may/28/maya-angelou-in-fifteen-quotes (Accessed 31 Jan 2024).

9. Brighton, L. (2019). *Romans Unplugged*. Wipf & Stock. (pp. 217-218)

10. Orr-Ewing, A. (2020). *Where is God in all the Suffering?* The Good Book Company. (p. 64)

11. McLaughlin, R. (17 June 2019) 'How Could a Loving God Allow So Much Suffering?' Chapter 11 of *Confronting Christianity*. Crossway Publishers 2019. Used by permission. biologos.org/articles/how-could-a-loving-god-allow-so-much-suffering

12. Hone, L. (2016). (p. 61)

13. Noel, J. (2015). (pp. 39, 93-107)

14. 'Ultra-marathon legend rediscovering life after paralysis' (30 May 2022). *1news*. www.1news.co.nz/2022/05/30/ultra-marathon-legend-rediscovering-life-after-paralysis/

15. Kierkegaard, S. (1843) in Ratcliffe, S. (Ed.). (2016). *Oxford Essential Quotations* (4 ed.). Oxford University Press. www.oxfordreference.com/display/10.1093/acref/9780191826719.001.0001/q-oro-ed4-00012432

16. Clifton, S. (2015). *Husbands Should Not Break*. Resource Publications. (p. 155)

17. 'Pequddah,' H6486. In Strong, J. *The New Strong's Exhaustive Concordance of the Bible*, Thomas Nelson, 1990. (p. 26)

18. F.B. Meyer Quotes. (n.d.). Goodreads.com. Retrieved February 24, 2025. From: www.goodreads.com/quotes/9808037-the-greatest-tragedy-of-life-is-not-unanswered-prayer-but

19. Dravecky, D. (1992). *When You Can't Come Back*. Harper Collins. Cited in *Christianity Today*, 38(2) (p. 39)

20. Nouwen, H. (2005). *The Dance of Life: Weaving sorrows and blessings into one joyful step*. (M. Ford, Ed.). Ave Maria Press. (p.163)

Chapter 7: I'm Broken But Can I Help You?

1. Havner, V. (n.d.). cited in Airey, J. (24 April 2022). StudioJake Media, studiojakemedia.com/2022/04/24/vance-havner-god-uses-broken-things/

2. Navani, A. (2023). 'Biologics in interventional spinal procedure: The past, the present, and the vision.' *Pain Physician*, 26(7). (pp. 775-785) www.painphysicianjournal.com/current/pdf?article=Nzc1OQ%3D%3D&journal=156

3. Keil, C.F., & Delitzsch, F. (1995). 'Isaiah 53.' *Keil and Delitzsch OT Commentary*. Bible Hub. biblehub.com/commentaries/kad/isaiah/53.htm

4. Walker, S., & Mulcahy, S. (Updated May 2022). 'Coping With Loss: The 7 Stages Of Grief.' Health Agenda Mental Health. HCF. www.hcf.com.au/health-agenda/body-mind/mental-health/moving-through-grief

5. Clifton, S. (2014). 'The dark side of healing: Toward a theology of wellbeing.' *Pneuma*, 36(2). (pp. 204-225)

6. Leo Tolstoy Quotes. (n.d.). Goodreads.com. Retrieved 28 October 2024. From: www.goodreads.com/quotes/36797-only-people-who-are-capable-of-loving-strongly-can-also

7. Frankl, V.E. (2014). (p. 76)

Chapter 8: Channels of Hope from the Weary

1. Flood, B. (10 November 2017). 'The locals proud to call Fordlands home.' *Rotorua Daily Post*. www.nzherald.co.nz/rotorua-daily-post/news/the-locals-proud-to-call-fordlands-home/XQ65GZKPFAHE7UHZ5XIUCEUQD4/
2. Hone, L. (2016). (pp. 108-110)
3. Nouwen, H. (2013). *Lifesigns: Intimacy, fecundity and ecstasy in Christian perspective*. Christian/Forum. (p. 18)
4. *Voice of Health*. (2023, 5 October). www.voiceofhealth.com.au/articles/how-you-can-utilise-your-lived-experience
5. 'Quote Origin: Comparison is the Thief of Joy.' (6 February 2021). quoteinvestigator.com/2021/02/06/thief-of-joy/

Chapter 9: Sharing the Beauty of 'God's own'

1. Leo, G. (2005). *Restoring Hope*. Self-published. (p. 43) thethinkingleader.org/restoring-hope
2. Williams, J. (10 July 2020) 'The Makingtrax Story.' *Vimeo* (07:36-07:38) vimeo.com/437013935. Also see https://internationalrafting.com/2021/02/jezza-williams-determination/
3. ibid. (06:36-06:58)

Chapter 10: Maybe Tomorrow Isn't So Bad After All!

1. Hone, L. (2016). (p. 179)
2. Nouwen, H. (7 January 2018). 'Living with Hope.' thecenterpalos.org/wp-content/uploads/2018/01/meditation010718.pdf
3. Wolf, J., & Wolf, K. (2020). (p. 72)
4. ibid. (p. 69)
5. Greig, P. (23 May 2019). '2. Adoration/ The Prayer Course/24-7 prayer.' 24-7 Prayer. Interview by Poppy Williams. *YouTube*. (10:06-11:32) www.youtube.com/watch?v=boklkec7NLE

6. Lewis, C.S. (1952). *Mere Christianity*. Chapter 10. (p. 143 of pdf). Available in various online formats here: www.fadedpage.com/showbook.php?pid=20150620

7. Brown, B. (2015). *Rising Strong*. Penguin Random House UK. (p. 202)

8. Wolf, J., & Wolf, K. (2020). (p. 193-194)

9. Mandela, N. (6 March 2000). 'Message to Healing & Reconciliation Service.' Nelson Rolihlahla Mandela 18 July 1918-5 December 2013.

Bible Versions Used

In addition to NIV (details on imprint page) the following versions have been quoted in this book:

Scripture quotations marked (NLT) are taken from the Holy Bible, New Living Translation, copyright ©1996, 2004, 2015 by Tyndale House Foundation. Used by permission of Tyndale House Publishers, Carol Stream, Illinois 60188. All rights reserved.

Scripture quotations marked (NRSV) are taken from the New Revised Standard Version Bible, copyright 1989, Division of Christian Education of the National Council of the Churches of Christ in the United States of America. Used by permission. All rights reserved.

Scripture quotations marked (NASB) are taken from the (NASB®) New American Standard Bible®, Copyright © 1960, 1971, 1977, 1995, 2020 by The Lockman Foundation. Used by permission. All rights reserved.

Scripture quotations marked (TLB) are taken from The Living Bible, copyright © 1971 by Tyndale House Foundation. Used by permission of Tyndale House Publishers, Carol Stream, Illinois 60188. All rights reserved.

Scripture quotations marked (NKJV) are taken from the New King James Version®. Copyright © 1982 by Thomas Nelson, Inc. Used by permission. All rights reserved.

Scripture quotations marked (ESV) are from The Holy Bible, English Standard Version®, copyright © 2001 by Crossway Bibles, a publishing ministry of Good News Publishers. Used by permission. All rights reserved.

Scripture quotations marked (CEV) are from the Contemporary English Version Copyright © 1991, 1992, 1995 by American Bible Society. Used by Permission.

About the Author

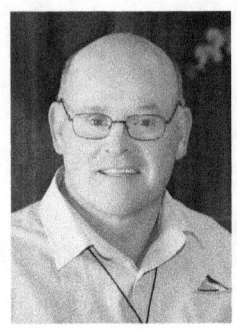 Rev. Timothy Lee serves as an itinerant Baptist pastor and preacher. He is a supervisor, chaplain, and an active leader and participant in several organisations and local community groups. Formerly a diesel mechanic in the agricultural industry, he grew up on a dairy farm and is very proud of his rural heritage. He is married to Jenny. They have two adult sons, a precious daughter-in-law, and a delightful young grandson.

www.ingramcontent.com/pod-product-compliance
Lightning Source LLC
Chambersburg PA
CBHW072334300426
44109CB00042B/1436